HANDBOOK OF METHODOLOGICAL CONCEPTS IN PERINATAL MEDICINE

OBSTETRICS AND GYNECOLOGY ADVANCES

Additional books in this series can be found on Nova's website
under the Series tab.

Additional e-books in this series can be found on Nova's website
under the e-book tab.

OBSTETRICS AND GYNECOLOGY ADVANCES

HANDBOOK OF METHODOLOGICAL CONCEPTS IN PERINATAL MEDICINE

EYAL SHEINER
EDITOR

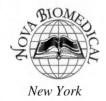

Nova Biomedical

New York

For permission to use material from this book please contact us:
Telephone 631-231-7269; Fax 631-231-8175
Web Site: http://www.novapublishers.com

NOTICE TO THE READER

The Publisher has taken reasonable care in the preparation of this book, but makes no expressed or implied warranty of any kind and assumes no responsibility for any errors or omissions. No liability is assumed for incidental or consequential damages in connection with or arising out of information contained in this book. The Publisher shall not be liable for any special, consequential, or exemplary damages resulting, in whole or in part, from the readers' use of, or reliance upon, this material. Any parts of this book based on government reports are so indicated and copyright is claimed for those parts to the extent applicable to compilations of such works.

Independent verification should be sought for any data, advice or recommendations contained in this book. In addition, no responsibility is assumed by the publisher for any injury and/or damage to persons or property arising from any methods, products, instructions, ideas or otherwise contained in this publication.

This publication is designed to provide accurate and authoritative information with regard to the subject matter covered herein. It is sold with the clear understanding that the Publisher is not engaged in rendering legal or any other professional services. If legal or any other expert assistance is required, the services of a competent person should be sought. FROM A DECLARATION OF PARTICIPANTS JOINTLY ADOPTED BY A COMMITTEE OF THE AMERICAN BAR ASSOCIATION AND A COMMITTEE OF PUBLISHERS.

Additional color graphics may be available in the e-book version of this book.

Library of Congress Cataloging-in-Publication Data

ISBN: 978-1-62081-252-5

Library of Congress Control Number: 2012933172

Published by Nova Science Publishers, Inc. † *New York*

CONTENTS

Preface   **vii**

Chapter 1   Perinatal Epidemiology   **1**
Eyal Sheiner

Chapter 2   Perinatal Events along the Perinatal Period:
Measures and Definitions   **9**
Ilana Shoham-Vardi

Chapter 3   Observational Study Design in Perinatal Epidemiology   **15**
Ilana Shoham-Vardi

Chapter 4   Randomized, Double-Blind, Placebo Controlled Trials:
Are they really the "Gold" Standard?   **25**
Anthony Odibo

Chapter 5   Data Analysis   **33**
Julia Harris and Eyal Sheiner

Chapter 6   Interpretation of Research Findings   **49**
Ilana Shoham-Vardi

Chapter 7   The Importance of Multivariable Analysis for Conducting
and Evaluating Research in Perinatology   **61**
Mitchell H. Katz

Chapter 8   Practical Guide for Data Analysis of Perinatal
Epidemiology by SPSS®   **77**
Amalia Levy

Chapter 9   Meta-Analyses   **107**
Hairong Xu and William D. Fraser

Chapter 10   Decision Analysis in Perinatal Medicine   **121**
William A. Grobman

Chapter 11   Ethics of Research on Perinatal Medicine   **135**
Frank A. Chervenak and Laurence B. McCullough

Index   **149**

PREFACE

This unique book stems from the "Textbook of perinatal epidemiology" and was conceived to satisfy the rising need for epidemiology-oriented clinicians. This book discusses methodological issues in perinatal epidemiology in a straightforward accessible manner. It gives a clear and comprehensive set of tools for practical research, and understanding perinatal epidemiology. This is an essential manual for the clinician for research in OB/Gyn. The book focuses on definitions, measures of disease frequency, prevalence and incidence of disease, sensitivity and specificity of studies, including examples from the perinatal world. It also discusses study design: observational or experimental, case controlled, randomized etc. Measure of association is discussed with examples (odds ratio, relative risk, attributed risk). Bias, statistical errors and sample size calculation, univariate analysis including examples and when to use parametric (Student t-test and Chi-squre test) as well as parametric tests are discussed too. An important chapter explains what multivariable analysis is and how to understand and construct a multiple logistic regression model. SPSS examples provide the reader the opportunity to repeat measurements, and understand the statistical analysis.

I would like to express my sincere gratitude for the authors who contributed excellent chapters.

Eyal Sheiner, Be'er-Sheva, 2012

In: Handbook of Methodological Concepts in Perinatal Medicine   ISBN: 978-1-62081-252-5
Editor: Eyal Sheiner   © 2013 Nova Science Publishers, Inc.

Chapter 1

PERINATAL EPIDEMIOLOGY

*Eyal Sheiner**

Departments of Obstetrics and Gynecology, Soroka University Medical Center, and the
Faculty of Health Sciences, Ben-Gurion University of the Negev, Beer-Sheva, Israel

WHAT IS EPIDEMIOLOGY?

Epidemiology is basically the study of an event (epidemic) that affects a population. Epidemiology deals with how disease, injury and clinical practice are distributed in populations and with the factors that influence or determine this distribution [1-3]. Many questions surround the epidemic of diseases: Who develops the disease? Where? When? How? Why did they develop the disease? [3]. Obviously, diseases are not randomly distributed in human populations, since there are several predisposing or protective characteristics (either genetic or acquired) for the disease [1]. Mostly, it seems that an interaction of genetic and environmental factors leads to the development of a disease [1]. Epidemiology also highlights the significance of disease control, i.e., measuring and identifying causes for diseases as well as interventions to improve health [3].

The specific objectives of epidemiology are to determine the following factors [1]:

1) *The cause of the disease:* e.g., human papillomavirus and cervical cancer. Infection with high-risk oncogenic HPV was found to be associated with precancerous lesions and cervical cancer [4].
2) *Prevalence*: the proportion of a population with a disease at a designated time, *and the incidence*, the rate of new cases during a period of time, *of the disease.* For example, cervical cancer is one of the most common types of cancer in women worldwide, with the highest rates observed in underdeveloped countries [4].
3) *Prognosis of the disease*

* Corresponding author: Eyal Sheiner, M.D, PhD, Department of Obstetrics and Gynecology, Soroka University Medical Center, P.O. Box 151, Faculty of Health Science, Ben-Gurion University of the Negev, Beer-Sheva, Israel. Tel 972-8-6403551, Fax 972-8-6403294, E-mail sheiner@bgu.ac.il.

4) *Effectiveness of preventive and/or therapeutic options:* e.g., advances in the understanding of the role of HPV in the etiology of high-grade cervical lesions [CIN 2/3] and cervical cancer have led to the development, evaluation and recommendation of two prophylactic HPV vaccines [4].

5) *Public policy related to disease prevention*

WHAT IS PERINATAL EPIDEMIOLOGY?

Events during pregnancy have a direct influence on both the health of the mother and the health of the child. Indeed, during pregnancy the obstetricians are dealing with two patients: the mother and the unborn child. Perinatal epidemiology deals with the epidemiology of the perinatal period, i.e., from 22 completed weeks of gestation to seven completed days after birth. Exposures of the mother, such as smoking and drug intake might have direct and indirect influences on the fetus. Moreover, several types of maternal exposures might have influence late into the adolescent life of the child. Perinatal epidemiology integrates care of both mother and child and incorporates the obstetrician's concern for the parturients with the pediatrician's concern for the newborn.

The improvement in perinatal health over the last decades is an impressive achievement of public health. Maternal and perinatal mortality rates have declined significantly over the years [5]. Nevertheless, statistics vary between countries. Awareness of the geographic gap in maternal mortality ratios led to the Safe Motherhood Initiative launched in 1987. The goal of this project was set at a 50–75% reduction in maternal mortality [5, 6]. Comparison of maternal mortality rates among populations must take into account different demopgraphic structures of the populations studied. Many parameters might bias this comparison, although age has the greatest influence upon mortality rates. For example, mortality rate in a low socioeconomic population may be surprisingly lower than in a high socioeconomic population only due to a much lower maternal age average in the low socioeconomic population.

Perinatal mortality rate is regarded as one of the major health indicators that reflect achievement in health in the referring communities. Perinatal mortality is the sum of early neonatal mortalities and late fetal deaths and the denominator for perinatal mortality rate is the number of live births or live births plus fetal deaths. Most cases are attributed to prematurity (figure 1) and accordingly are associated with low birth weight (figure 2). For this reason, perinatal mortality rates reach 85% before 24-25 weeks of gestation, and are roughly 95% in newborns weighing less than 500 grams. On the other hand, mortality rises to 15% in fetuses with birth weights greater than 5500 grams.

Medical litigation and concern regarding fetal well-being have, however, brought cesarean delivery to an epidemic. Cesarean delivery (CD) rates have risen constantly in the last decade. Contributing factors are particular practice patterns and patient preferences, as well as the decrease in the rate of vaginal births after cesarean (VBAC) and decrease in vaginal births of breech pregnancies [7]. The steady increase in cesarean deliveries over the years is illustrated in figures 3 and 4. The rates of CD changed from an average of 10% between 1985 and 1989 to over 20% in 2006. Figure 4 reflects trends for more births and more CDs over the years, and accordingly the percentage of CDs increase dramatically (total CDs in all years equals 100%).

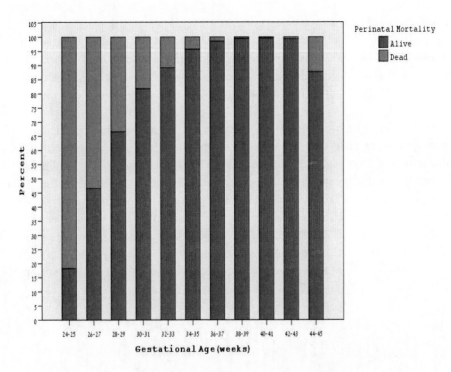

Figure 1. Perinatal mortality according to the gestational age; data from Soroka University Medical Center.

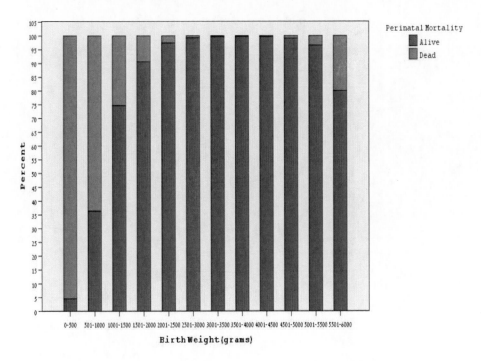

Figure 2. Perinatal mortality according to birthweight; data from Soroka University Medical Center.

PREVENTION STRATEGIES

Epidemiologic analysis is a complex process. First, we have to determine if an association exists between exposure and disease (i.e., obesity and diabetes), and whether it is a causal association [1]. Descriptive statistics is the first step: once variables have been defined and measured, we need to draw conclusions from the data collected on these variables. Nevertheless, we must make sure that the data are valid and the differences are real. This is the time to examine potential biases, interactions and control for confounders using a multivariable analysis.

If we can identify high risk groups, we can move from observations to preventive actions and direct preventive efforts such as screening programs (i.e., Papanicolaou [Pap] smear: screening programs have significantly reduced the incidence and death rates in the Western world from cervical cancer) [8] or remove the risk factor if possible (i.e., smoking). Importantly, there are modifiable risk factors (such as obesity), but there are risk factors such as age (which can be associated with infertility, for example) that are not modifiable.

Two possible methods of prevention are a population-based approach vs. a high-risk approach [1]. It is difficult to reach a consensus regarding screening approaches since it is a matter of cost effectiveness as well. A measure that will be applied to the entire population must be inexpensive and minimally invasive [1].

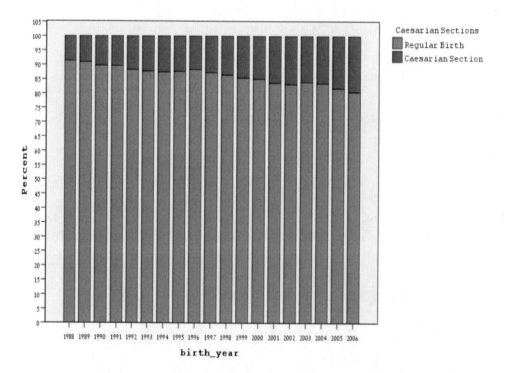

Figure 3. Cesarean section rates over the years (% for each year); data from Soroka University Medical Center.

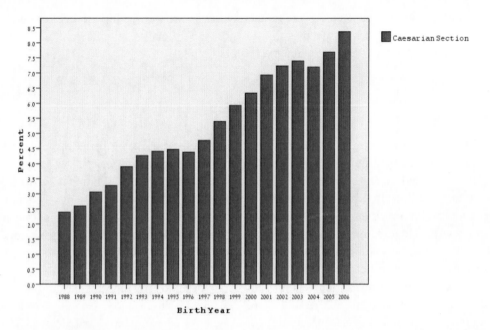

Figure 4. Distribution of all cesarean section cases over the years (% of total cesarean deliveries); data from Soroka University Medical Center.

Screening for gestational diabetes mellitus (GDM) is performed using the glucose challenge test (GCT). Screening recommendations range from the inclusion of all pregnant women (universal) to the exclusion of all women except those with highly specific risk factors (selective) including: age (>25 years); obesity (body mass index [BMI]>30 Kg/m^2; ethnicity (Hispanic, Native American, Asian American, African-American); family history (first-degree relative with diabetes); and previous GDM or large-for-gestational-age infant. Moreover, the cut-off value of the GCT matters as well: a value of 140 mg/dL will identify 80% of women with GDM, while a lower cut-off of 130 mg/dL will identify more than 80% of women with GDM (increased *sensitivity*, which measures the proportion of actual positives that are correctly identified as such, but decreased *specificity*, which measures the proportion of negatives that are correctly identified). In Israel, screening for GDM as well as the triple test (genetic screening for Down syndrome) are offered to all pregnant women.

Three types of preventions exist:

- Primary prevention: Action taken to prevent the occurrence of the disease, such as folic acid for prevention of neural tube defects [9].
- Secondary prevention: Identification of a population in the pre-clinical phase of the disease, i.e., they do not yet have clinical symptoms [1]. In such cases, treatment is easier and more effective, and might prevent mortality. The effectiveness of anticoagulant therapy and thromboprophylaxis in patients with thrombophilia might serve as an example for secondary prevention.
- Tertiary prevention: Preventing complications in patients who have already developed signs and symptoms of the disease in order to prevent end-stage complications (such as renal failure in patients with type 2 diabetes with proper treatment) [1].

Studies regarding the health of the mother and fetus are well within the field of perinatal epidemiology, which has evolved into a major sub-specialty of epidemiology and an important component of perinatal medicine [10,11].

IN THIS BOOK

The book focuses on epidemiology and methodological issues including definitions, measures of disease frequency, prevalence and incidence of diseases, sensitivity and specificity of studies, and includes examples from the perinatal world. Perinatal events along the perinatal period are discussed in details. Multivariable analysis is essential to the study of perinatology. An important chapter explains what multivariable analysis is, why is it needed, what types of multivariable analyses are commonly used in perinatal research, how to understand and construct a multiple logistic regression model, how well the model predicts outcome, and whether the model is reliable.

SPSS examples provide the reader with the opportunity to repeat measurements and understand the statistical analysis. Other chapters discuss study design. While the randomized, double-blind placebo-controlled design has come to be regarded as the "gold standard" to which other designs of clinical research should be compared [12-14], it surely has limitations. A chapter dealing with RCT (randomized controlled trials) highlights the advantages, but also sounds a note of caution in the conduct and interpretation of the results of these trials. A chapter regarding decision analysis (i.e., a quantitative analysis that combines information, using a formal stepwise process, in an attempt to aid the process of decision making) follows. Decision analysis is an interesting type of study design that can provide useful insights, and is particularly helpful in circumstances in which an interventional or observational study design cannot provide the required information needed to differentiate between different tests or therapies.

Meta-analysis is a study that combines the results of several studies that address a set of related research hypotheses. Synthesis of available evidence remains essential for good clinical practice. A systematic review is a slightly different form of research that provides a summary of medical reports, using explicit methods to search, critically appraise and synthesize the published or unpublished evidence concerning a specific clinical question. Quantitative systematic review, or meta-analysis, combines different studies to produce an overall effect estimate of a specific treatment using explicit statistical techniques. The role of systematic reviews and meta-analyses has been increasingly endorsed in the practice of evidence-based decision making. The chapter provides an overview of basic and quantitative methods and issues needed to be considered for the conduct of a meta-analysis.

At the end of the book, ethics in perinatal research is discussed: Less than optimal treatment of pregnant and fetal patients may lead to serious clinical sequelae. Clinical concerns lend urgency to the need to conduct well-designed clinical investigations of interventions with pregnant women and fetuses to improve the outcomes of perinatal medicine. Investigators in perinatal research must address and responsibly manage ethical challenges related to the protection of both the pregnant patient's and fetal patient's health-related interests. The chapter identifies the international consensus that has formed on ethics of perinatal research, focusing on research of fetal interventions and obstetric ultrasound.

REFERENCES

[1]   Gordis L. *Epidemiology*. Philadelphia: Saunders, Elsevier, 2009.

[2]   Jekel F, James., Katz L, David., Elmore G, Joann., Wild M, Dorothea. *Epidemiology, Biostatistics, and Preventive Medicine*. Philadelphia: Saunders, Elsevier, 2007.

[3]   Webb P, Bain C, Pirozzo S. *Essential Epidemiology*. Cambridge, UK: Cambridge University Press, 2005.

[4]   Oaknin A, Barretina MP. Human papillomavirus vaccine and cervical cancer prevention. *Clin Transl Oncol* 2008;10:804-11.

[5]   Schneid-Kofman N, Sheiner E. Frustration from not achieving the expected reduction in maternal mortality. *Arch Gynecol Obstet* 2008;277:283-4.

[6]   Freedman LP, Graham WJ, Brazier E, et al. Practical lessons from global safe motherhood initiatives: time for a new focus on implementation. *Lancet* 2007;370:1383-91.

[7]   Menacker F, Declercq E, Macdorman MF. Cesarean delivery: background, trends, and epidemiology. *Semin Perinatol* 2006;30:235-41.

[8]   Lowy DR, Solomon D, Hildesheim A, Schiller JT, Schiffman M. Human papillomavirus infection and the primary and secondary prevention of cervical cancer. *Cancer* 2008;113:1980-93.

[9]   Cordero JF, Do A, Berry RJ. Review of interventions for the prevention and control of folate and vitamin B12 deficiencies. *Food Nutr Bull* 2008;29:S188-95.

[10] Bracken B, Michael. *Perinatal Epidemiology*. Oxford: Oxford University Press, 1984.

[11] Sheiner E. Textbook of Perinatal Epidemiology. Nova Science Publishers, NY, 2010.

[12] Beswick AD, Rees K, West RR, et al. Improving uptake and adherence in cardiac rehabilitation: literature review. *J Adv Nurs* 2005;49:538-55.

[13] Cook NR, Cohen J, Hebert PR, Taylor JO, Hennekens CH. Implications of small reductions in diastolic blood pressure for primary prevention. *Arch Intern Med* 1995;155:701-9.

[14] Hennekens CH, Buring JE, Hebert PR. Implications of overviews of randomized trials. *Stat Med* 1987;6:397-409.

In: Handbook of Methodological Concepts in Perinatal Medicine   ISBN: 978-1-62081-252-5
Editor: Eyal Sheiner   © 2013 Nova Science Publishers, Inc.

Chapter 2

PERINATAL EVENTS ALONG THE PERINATAL PERIOD: MEASURES AND DEFINITIONS

*Ilana Shoham-Vardi**

Department of Epidemiology and Health Services Evaluation, Faculty of Health
Sciences, Ben Gurion University of the Negev, Beer Sheva, Israel

1. THE TIME FRAMES OF THE PERINATAL AND NEONATAL PERIODS

According to latest version of the International Classification of Disease and Causes of Death (ICD-10) [1], the World Health Organization (WHO) defines the perinatal period as the time that "commences at 22 completed weeks (154 days) of gestation (the time when birth weight is normally 500 g), and ends seven completed days after birth". The last seven days of the perinatal period overlap the first week of the neonatal period, which ends at 28 completed days after birth. This overlapping period is known as the early neonatal period, while the last three weeks of the neonatal period are known as the late neonatal period.

Events occurring around conception and during the early stages of pregnancy are outside the perinatal period, which begins at the lowest threshold for fetal survival. As medical technology has progressed in the last 20 years, the threshold of fetal survival has been lowered, but current opinion holds that the threshold for survival is 23–24 weeks of gestation [2]. Differences exist between countries regarding the legal definition of the lowest limit of the perinatal period [3]. These differences affect medical practices regarding treatment of very premature infants, as well as international comparisons and assessment of time trends of perinatal statistics.

The lowest limit of this time frame is set in terms of gestational age, while the upper limit is set by the newborn age, regardless of gestational age. The simultaneous use of these two time scales has recently been addressed as a methodological issue in perinatal epidemiology [4]. Thus, a live birth can, by definition (see below), occur at any time in pregnancy, while the outcome of pregnancy resulting in a non live birth is classified by WHO according to the

---
* Tel +972-8-6477453; Fax +972-8-6477638; Email: vilana@bgu.ac.il.

length of gestation. Pregnancy outcomes in early pregnancy (<22 weeks of gestation) are defined as outside of the perinatal period, since such pregnancies very rarely end in a live birth. The most common outcome at that stage of pregnancy is "early pregnancy loss", which often goes unrecognized. In studies with careful monitoring by daily urine samples of women trying to conceive, it was shown that about one-third of conceptions are not carried to delivery and two-thirds of those losses occur before they are recognized [5].

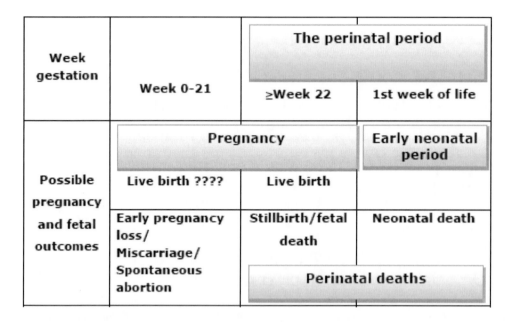

Figure 1. Gestational, perinatal and neonatal periods and outcomes of pregnancy.

2. PREGNANCY OUTCOMES IN THE PERINATAL PERIOD

2.1. Definitions

- Live birth: The WHO defines a live birth as "the complete expulsion or extraction from its mother of a product of conception, irrespective of the duration of the pregnancy, which, after such separation, breathes or shows any other evidence of life, such as beating of the heart, pulsation of the umbilical cord, or definite movement of voluntary muscles, whether or not the umbilical cord has been cut or the placenta is attached; each product of such a birth is considered liveborn" [1]. In 1992, a revision to this definition was made in the United States. Two main changes were made: (1) Spontaneous fetal deaths were distinguished from induced terminations of pregnancy and excluded from fetal death statistics, and (2) a more restricted description was added to the term "signs of life": heartbeats are to be distinguished from transient cardiac contractions and respirations are to be distinguished from fleeting respiratory efforts or gasps [6].
- Fetal death: When a pregnancy over 22 weeks of gestation does not result in a live birth, the outcome of pregnancy is termed fetal death or stillbirth, defined by WHO

as "death prior to the complete expulsion or extraction from its mother of a product of conception, irrespective of the duration of pregnancy; the death is indicated by the fact that after such separation the fetus does not breathe or show any other evidence of life, such as beating of the heart, pulsation of the umbilical cord, or definite movement of voluntary muscles" [1].

- Neonatal death: A death of a live-born during the first 28 completed days of life. The neonatal period is subdivided into early neonatal, the first seven days of life; and the late neonatal period, 7–28 completed days of life. Early neonatal deaths are counted as perinatal deaths.
- Perinatal death: Fetal deaths + early neonatal deaths
- Infant death: Death of a live-born infant during the first year of life, including neonatal deaths and post-neonatal deaths. Only deaths in the first week of life are counted as perinatal deaths.

2.2. Reporting Requirements

It is important to note that neither WHO definition of live birth nor those of fetal death are dependent on gestational age. The reporting requirements (and the vital statistics of these outcomes), however, are defined by gestational age and/or birth weight. WHO recommends that all fetuses and infants weighing at least 500 g at birth should be included in the statistics whether alive or dead. Fetal deaths occurring before 22 completed weeks of gestation or weighing less than 500 g are to be reported separately as *miscarriages or spontaneous abortions*. Moreover, for international comparisons, WHO sets the limit of reporting at 28 weeks gestation and/or 1000 g at birth.

2.3. International Comparison of Definitions of Perinatal Events

The US reporting requirements, which were revised in 1995, state that all spontaneous fetal deaths (to be distinguished from induced abortions) weighing 350 grams or more—or, if weight is unknown, having completed 20 weeks of gestation—should be reported as fetal deaths [6]. These requirements, however, vary among countries [3] and in the US between states [3,7]. In the National Vital Statistics Reports of the 2004 perinatal mortality data [7], two different definitions of perinatal mortality are used: Definition I (generally used for international comparisons): fetal deaths of 28 weeks of gestation or more and infant deaths under 7 days; Definition II: fetal deaths of 20 weeks of gestation or more and infant deaths under 28 days.

In Australia since 2006, the lowest limit for reporting fetal deaths was set at 20 weeks or 400 grams [8]. In the UK, the lowest limit for reporting fetal deaths is 24 completed weeks of gestation [9]. An effort has been made by members of the European Union through the Euro-Peristat project to create uniform European standards to report perinatal information. In a recent report summarizing the project [10], the lower limit for calculating perinatal mortality was set at 28 weeks of gestation.

2.4. Measures of Perinatal Mortality

There are several measures of perinatal mortality that are commonly used in vital statistics. Table 1 shows how the measures are calculated in terms of numerator and denominators. All measures are usually expressed per 1000 either live births or total births (including live births + fetal deaths), usually in a year, in a defined population.

Table 1. Commonly used measures of perinatal mortality

Measure	Numerator	Denominator	10^x
Fetal death ratio	Fetal deaths	Live births	1000
Fetal death rate	Fetal deaths	Total births (live births+fetal deaths)	1000
Early neonatal mortality rate	Early neonatal deaths	Live births	1000
Perinatal mortality rate	Fetal deaths + Early neonatal deaths	Total births (live births + fetal deaths)	1000

3. DEFINITIONS OF GESTATIONAL PERIODS

The period of gestation is traditionally divided into three periods: preterm, term and post-term. Table 2 shows the WHO definitions of these periods.

Table 2. Division of the gestational period according to WHO definition

Pre-term	Before 37 completed weeks (less than 259 days) of gestation
Term	Completed 37 weeks –up to 41 weeks (259–293 days) of gestation
Post-term	42 completed weeks or more (294 days or more) of gestation

Crucial to these definitions is the timing of conception and estimating the length of time between conception and any event during pregnancy, i.e., determining gestational age. According to the WHO definition, the duration of gestation is measured from the first day of the last normal menstrual period, which is counted as day zero. Gestational age is expressed in completed days or completed weeks; thus, week 1 of gestation begins on day 7 (after completion of gestational week zero), and is completed on day 13. When information on last menstrual period is unavailable or unreliable, gestational age is determined by other means. The most widely-used method in developed countries is an ultrasound assessment during the first 20 weeks of pregnancy, when the inter-pregnancy variance in fetal size is negligible.

Several studies compared pregnancy dating in cohorts of pregnant women whose pregnancy was assessed by reliable information about last menstrual period (LMP) and by ultrasound during the first 20 weeks of gestation. Systematic differences were noted between the two most common methods of dating [11]. Ultrasound dating, which is based on comparing fetal measurements to standard fetal week-specific growth distributions, tends to slightly underestimate the gestational age of small fetuses, resulting in overestimate of preterm births, especially in population groups with smaller fetuses [12]. A recent study, however, has shown that rates of both preterm and post-term estimates were higher if dating was LMP-based in comparison to ultrasound-based dating [13]. LMP vs. ultrasound estimates were, respectively, 8.7% vs. 7.9% preterm (<37 weeks), 81.2% vs. 91.0% term (37–41 weeks), and 10.1% vs. 1.1% post-term (≥42 weeks). Studies based on artificial reproductive technologies-conceived pregnancies provide a unique opportunity to study the quality of dating methods, as the date of conception is not based on recall of LMP but rather on the actual date of fertilization. A study done on such a cohort revealed that inaccuracies in data entry are another source of error causing misclassification of gestational age [14]. Errors in gestational age estimates were also noted in a study done on a large cohort in Sweden [15]. Such errors, if likely to occur in specific populations more than in other populations, may bias our estimates of differences among population groups and trends in preterm births [16].

4. DEFINITIONS OF BIRTH WEIGHTS

Birth weight is the first weight of the fetus or newborn obtained after birth. Table 3 presents the division of the gestational period according to WHO definitions. The definitions of "low", "very low" and "extremely low" birth weight overlap (i.e., "low" includes "very low" and "extremely low", while "very low" includes "extremely low").

Table 3. Classification of birth weight according to WHO definition

Low birth weight	Less than 2500 grams (up to and including 2499 gram
Very low birth weight	Less than 1500 grams (up to and including 1499 grams)
Extremely low birth weight	Less than 1000 grams (up to and including 999 grams)

REFERENCES

[1]   http://www.icd10.ch/ebook/FRetENetGe_OMSetDIMDI_FR/ICD10_Volume_2_Par_5.7.1.asp.

[2]   Pignotti MS, Donzelli G. Perinatal care at the threshold of viability: an international comparison of practical guidelines for the treatment of extremely preterm births. *Pediatrics.* 2008; 121(1):e193-8.

[3]   Nguyen RHN, Wilcox AJ Terms in reproductive and perinatal epidemiology: II, Perinatal terms. 2005; *J Epidemiology Community Health* 59:9196-921.

[4]   Joseph KS. Incidence based measures of birth, growth restriction, and death can free perinatal epidemiology from erroneous concepts of risk. *J Clinical Epidemiol* 2004; 57:889-897.

[5]   Wang X, Chen C, Wang L, Chen D, Guang W, French J. Conception, early pregnancy loss, and time to clinical pregnancy: a population-based prospective study. *Fertil Steril.* 2003;79:577-84.

[6]   *National Center for Health Statistics.* Model state vital statistics act and model state vital statistics regulations. Washington: Public Health Service. 1995.

[7]   MacDorman MF, Munson ML, Kirmeyer S. Fetal and perinatal mortality, United States, 2004. *Natl Vital Stat Rep.* 2007;56:1-19.

[8]   *http://www.health.nsw.gov.au/policies/pd/2006/PD2006_006.html.*

[9]   *Office for National Statistics. Mortality Statistics:* Childhood, infant and perinatal. Review of the national Statistician on death in England and Wales, 2006 (Series DH3. no 39).

[10] *European Perinatal Health Report. 2008.* http://www.europeristat.com/publications/european-perinatal-health-report.shtml.

[11] 11.Lynch CD, Zhang J.The research implications of the selection of a gestational age estimation method. *Paediatr Perinat Epidemiol.* 2007;21 Suppl 2:86-96.

[12] Yang H, Kramer MS, Platt RW, Blondel B, Bréart G, Morin I, Wilkins R, Usher R.How does early ultrasound scan estimation of gestational age lead to higher rates of preterm birth? *Am J Obstet Gynecol.* 2002 ;186:433-7.

[13] Dietz PM, England LJ, Callaghan WM, Pearl M, Wier ML, Kharrazi M. A comparison of LMP-based and ultrasound-based estimates of gestational age using linked California livebirth and prenatal screening records. *Paediatr Perinat Epidemiol.* 2007;21 Suppl 2:62-71.

[14] Callaghan WM, Schieve LA, Dietz PM.Gestational age estimates from singleton births conceived using assisted reproductive technology. *Paediatr Perinat Epidemiol.* 2007;21 Suppl 2:79-85.

[15] Haglund B:Birthweight distributions by gestational age: comparison of LMP-based and ultrasound-based estimates of gestational age using data from the Swedish Birth Registry. *Paediatr Perinat Epidemiol.* 2007 ;21 Suppl 2:72-8.

[16] Qin C, Dietz PM, England LJ, Martin JA, Callaghan WM.Effects of different data-editing methods on trends in race-specific preterm delivery rates, United States, 1990-2002. *Paediatr Perinat Epidemiol.* 2007;21 Suppl 2:41-9.

In: Handbook of Methodological Concepts in Perinatal Medicine   ISBN: 978-1-62081-252-5
Editor: Eyal Sheiner   © 2013 Nova Science Publishers, Inc.

Chapter 3

OBSERVATIONAL STUDY DESIGN IN PERINATAL EPIDEMIOLOGY

Ilana Shoham-Vardi

Department of Epidemiology and Health Services Utilization Faculty
of Health Sciences, Ben-Gurion University of the Negev,
Beer Sheva, Israel

DEFINITIONS

- Cohort: A group of people who share a common characteristic within a defined period.
- Cohort study: A comparison of incidence of a defined clinical outcome in exposed and unexposed persons.
- Case-control study: A comparison of prevalence of exposure in persons with a defined disease or clinical condition (cases) with prevalence of exposure in persons without the disease or condition (controls).

INTRODUCTION

Epidemiological studies are designed to test hypotheses regarding the etiology of disease by studying the patterns and strength of associations between exposures and defined health outcomes, and to provide the most valid estimate of this association. Perinatal epidemiology is mainly focused on the examination of exposures that are hypothesized to affect perinatal outcomes. There is, however, a growing body of research that focuses on perinatal events and fetal environment as exposures that affect health outcomes later in life [1,2]. This chapter will review the most common study designs used in observational perinatal epidemiology.

COHORT STUDIES

Cohort studies compare incidence of a defined clinical outcome in exposed and unexposed persons. Study participants are assessed at baseline to determine (1) their eligibility status according to predefined inclusion and exclusion criteria and (2) their exposure status to hypothesized risk factor(s). Disease occurrence is monitored and incidence rates are computed for the exposed and unexposed groups and compared. The most common measures of association in cohort studies are risk ratios or relative risks.

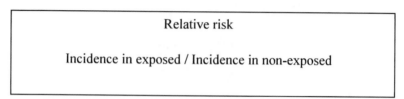

Cohort studies can be either prospective or retrospective (see below), but in all cohort studies the measure of disease occurrence is incidence: i.e., the new occurrence of disease in persons free of disease at the time exposure is assessed.

Table 1. Cohort Studies Design

Time 1 (Baseline)	1. Determining participation eligibility (inclusion/exclusion criteria) 2. Measure of exposure to hypothesized risk factor/s (exposed/unexposed)
Time 1–Time 2	Follow-up period
Time 2	Measure of disease occurrence

Prospective Cohort Studies

In this type of study, the researcher defines a cohort in which incidence of disease is to be assessed. After the cohort has been defined by meeting eligibility criteria, exposure status of all cohort members is measured and participants are classified into exposed and unexposed. After the baseline assessment, the researcher actually follows in real time the disease experience of exposed and unexposed study participants and determines the incidence of disease at some defined point of time in the future.

One of the most problematic issues in conducting prospective cohort studies is the length of time between the assessment of exposure status and the occurrence of disease. The EPIC study [3], for example, is a large multi-center study designed to investigate the relation between diet, nutritional and metabolic characteristics, various lifestyle factors and the risk of cancer. It is expected to conduct lifetime follow-up on about 400,000 middle-aged participants. In perinatal epidemiology, where the variable of interest often is the outcome of pregnancy, the follow-up period is relatively short, allowing studies of the effects of prenatal exposures and pregnancy outcomes to be designed as prospective cohort studies. In a study conducted in Sweden, 866,188 women with singleton pregnancy were followed from the first antenatal visit to delivery. The study showed that mothers with chronic hypertension had an increased risk of perinatal mortality of their male, but not of their female, offspring [4]. Another example is a study showing an association between elevated free fatty acids measured at 30 weeks of pregnancy and the risk for preterm delivery [5], or a study conducted in Denmark on large cohort of pregnant women showing that level of high stress assessed at week 30 is associated with an increased risk for stillbirth [6]. In all of these studies, the length of follow-up needed was relatively short.

Studies of "time to pregnancy" aiming at detection of factors associated with the likelihood of conception and carrying a pregnancy to delivery are usually conducted as prospective cohort studies. A cohort of 443 women with pelvic inflammatory disease (PID) was followed up for 84 months to assess rates of pregnancy and recurrence of disease. Exposure was defined as the highest tertile level of antibody titers to chlamydia measured in the final follow-up year. The investigators concluded that the level of antibodies to *C. trachomatis* was associated with reduced likelihood of pregnancy and elevated risk of recurrent PID [7].

As the interest in the fetal origin of adult disease has been growing in recent years, several large-scale prospective cohort studies have been carried out to test hypotheses regarding the risks associated with various fetal environments and perinatal events. The Generation R Study is a study based on a cohort of 9,778 mothers in the Netherlands designed to assess characteristics and events in fetal life and early postnatal life that impact growth, development and health status in childhood and young adulthood [8]. The Jerusalem Perinatal Study has been following a population-based cohort of 80,936 offspring born in Jerusalem between 1964 and 1976. This study has demonstrated, among other findings, that birth weight is inversely associated with the risk of mortality in male adults age 15+ [9]. About 55,000 pregnancies resulting in live births comprised the cohort in the Collaborative Perinatal Project, which was originally designed to study the causes of neurological defects. Children were actively followed until age 7–8 years. A recent report has suggested an increased risk of childhood cancers in children with a documented birthmark, as compared with children with no birthmarks [10].

Retrospective Cohort Studies

Cohort studies can be conducted in a retrospective way when information about exposure had been collected for an entire cohort in the past. The researcher can use this information at a later point when all or some incident events had already occurred. These studies depend on valid documentation of the exposure of interest in the past; thus, they can be carried out in a relatively short time, as the period between exposure and disease occurrence had already elapsed at the time the study is carried out.

This study design is frequently used in perinatal epidemiology where prenatal information is routinely collected and documented in a uniform way for large cohorts of women. Availability of this kind of information allows testing new hypotheses about risk factors and incidence of disease without starting a new cohort study. It is especially useful when rare exposures are studied. A retrospective cohort study was conducted to examine the association between gestational weight gain and perinatal outcomes in women with gestational diabetes mellitus [11]. The cohort comprised all women (n=31,074) participating in a program for women with gestational diabetes in California between 2001 and 2004.

Information about gestational weight gain was available for all program participants, and was retrieved from medical records after all study participants had already given birth. The study found that women who had gestational weight gain above the Institute of Medicine (IOM) guidelines had a higher risk of undesirable outcomes including preterm delivery, having macrosomic neonates, and cesarean delivery, while women who gained weight below IOM recommendations were more likely to have small-for-gestational-age neonates.

A large number of studies were conducted in Soroka University Medical Center (SUMC), Beer Sheva, Israel, which is the only tertiary hospital serving the entire population of Southern Israel (about 13,000 birth annually), and where prenatal information is available for population-based nonselective cohorts of births. Most women in the area attend maternal and child clinics for prenatal care. Thus, prenatal information is available to almost all women and is part of the computerized database of all birth records. Such a setting allows for the study of rather rare exposures, such as deep venous thrombosis [12] and Familial Mediterranean Fever during pregnancy [13], both of which were found to be associated with risk for preterm births.

Retrospective cohort studies can be conducted by linking databases such as the Swedish Conscript Study, where birth information from the Swedish Birth Register was individually linked to the Swedish Conscript Register, resulting in a cohort of 168,068 males. This study revealed that males born small for gestational age were at increased risk of subnormal intellectual performance compared to males born with adequate weight for gestational age [14].

Comparison of Prospective and Retrospective Cohort Studies

Cohort studies examine the effect of exposure on incidence of disease. The difference between these two types of studies is the way information becomes available to the researcher, but not in the way information had originally been collected. In both types of studies, exposure information is recorded before disease occurrence. Prospective cohort studies are also called concurrent cohort studies, as the follow-up is conducted in real time, while in retrospective cohort studies, also called historical cohort studies, the follow-up period had been completed at the time the study was initiated. Sometimes retrospective studies are the first stage in a multistage study and are continued with an active prospective follow-up for an additional period of time for studying participants who had not developed the disease at the time the retrospective study had been performed.

CASE-CONTROL STUDIES

When the disease of interest is rare, a cohort study might not be an efficient study design, as it requires following large number of people for long periods of time. In case-control studies, we compare persons with a defined disease or clinical condition (cases), and persons without the disease or condition (controls). We then measure retrospectively past exposures, which are hypothesized to be related to the disease. Our hypothesis is that exposures which are risk factors for the disease will be more prevalent among cases than among controls. Since exposure information is collected retrospectively, after the disease status is known, the evidence of an association between exposure and disease is considered to be weaker than that obtained form cohort studies. Since in case-control studies we cannot measure incidence, relative risks or risk ratios cannot be computed. The most common measure of association used in case-control studies is Exposure Odds Ratio (the ratio of exposure odds in cases relative to odds of exposure in controls).

	DISEASE STUATUS	
EXPOSURE	CASES	CONTROLS
Present	a	c
Absent	b	d
Total	a+b	c+d

Odds of Exposure among cases: a / (a+b) : b/ (a+b) = a / b

Odds of Exposure among controls: c / (c+d) : d/ (c+d) = c / d

Exposure Odds Ratio

$$(a / b) : (c / d) = (a \times d) / (b \times c)$$

It can be shown that case-control studies that are properly conducted, i.e., the cases are representative of persons with the disease and controls of persons without the disease, and we study a rare disease, the exposure odds ratio (OR) is a good estimate of the relative risk, which would have been obtained from a cohort study.

The main advantages of case-control studies is that they are usually smaller and can be conducted in a relatively shorter time and consequently require less resources than cohort studies. However, case-control studies, more than cohort studies, are considered to be prone to selection and information biases (see Chapter 6). In perinatal epidemiology, case-control studies are usually conducted when a rare clinical condition is investigated. For example, a national case-control study was conducted in France to assess the role of ethnicity and nationality in maternal mortality, which is a very rare occurrence in France [15]. The study comprised a total of 267 cases of maternal deaths from 1996 to 2001 and a representative sample (n = 13,186) of women who gave birth in 1998 as controls. The study found that women from sub-Saharan Africa and women from Asia, North and South America were more likely to die postpartum than women born in France (odds ratios were 5.5 and 3.3, respectively).

The choice of appropriate controls is the major challenge in case-control studies. Controls should be chosen from the same population that gave rise to the cases. For example, if cases were identified through prenatal clinics, controls should be chosen from women attending the same clinics but without the condition ; if cases were identified at birth, controls should also be identified at birth at the same hospitals, etc. Case-control studies often choose more than one control per case. This is done to increase the statistical power of the study. There are case-control studies that use different control groups which allow controlling for different confounders, or to test a hypothesis under different conditions. A population-based case-control study is being conducted in Hungary to study risk factors for birth defects. In a recently published study, all cases (n=111) of isolated congenital cataract were compared to

111 matched controls without the defect to 37,837 population controls without any defects and to 22,744 malformed controls with other nonocular abnormalities [16].

Matched Case-control Studies

In order to make case-control studies more efficient, controls are sometimes not randomly chosen from the non-diseased population but are chosen to match cases in one or more characteristics. The matching factors are usually known risk factors that have already been shown to be associated with the disease. Matching such factor(s) reduces the variability in the study population, but creates a situation in which controls are not a representative sample of all non-diseased persons, and this needs to be accounted for when conclusions are drawn from a matched case-control study. The decision to use matching in choosing controls should be made after consideration of the advantages and disadvantages of matching in each particular study.

In a recently published case-control study of vascular dysfunction and cardiovascular risk factors in mothers of growth-restricted offspring, cases were 28 women with infants born at term below the 5th percentile of weight for gestational age and controls were 29 mothers of term infants born at the 25th–90th percentile of weight for gestational age [17]. Controls were matched to cases by age at index pregnancy, parity, body mass index and gestational age at booking prenatal care, and gestational age at delivery. Cases were found to have significantly higher proportions of perturbation of metabolic and vascular function than controls 3–4 years after the index birth. In the latter study, intensive and expensive testing was done that would not be feasible in a larger study. Matching helped to reduce the number of participants needed for the analysis, as many possible confounders were eliminated. While matching can make a study more efficient, it can introduce a selection bias if any of the matching factors is too closely associated with the exposure of interest; this is called "over-matching", and may cause an underestimation of a true difference between cases and controls. For example, if one of the cardiovascular risk factors studied were too closely associated with parity, which was one of the matching factors, the difference observed in the study between cases and controls might be smaller than that in the target population because the controls that were chosen through the matching process were too similar to the cases.

Controls can be individually matched to cases, i.e., each case will have its matched control/s (individual matching), or the control group can be chosen in such a way that the frequency distribution of the matching factors is similar in both study groups. When individual matching is employed, procedures appropriate for non-independent samples statistical analysis should be used.

Special Designs of Case-control Studies in Perinatal Epidemiology

The most frequently special design case-controls studies used in perinatal epidemiology, are the "nested case-control" design and the "case cohort" designs [18].

Nested Case-Control Studies

In these case-control studies, the two study groups are drawn from a large cohort study when a sufficient number of cases have occurred. Controls are drawn from the rest, non-diseased cohort members. A nested case-control study was conducted in Sweden to investigate prenatal, perinatal and neonatal risk factors for neuroblastoma [19]. Cases (n=245) were identified through the Swedish Cancer Register. The list was linked with the Swedish Medical Birth Register, and five living controls per case were randomly selected from the birth registry, matched by gender and age. The researchers concluded that neuroblastoma in infancy, but not with diagnoses at one year or older, are associated with some markers of prenatal, perinatal and neonatal distress. In this study, information about exposure was obtained from available medical records. In other nested case-control studies, this design is used when information regarding exposure is unavailable and needs to be collected for both cases and controls. Drawing the cases and controls from a large representative cohort may reduce the potential selection bias, which is often an issue in case-control studies.

Case Cohort Design

When cases are drawn from an ongoing cohort, controls can be drawn from the "risk set", i.e., all of the population at risk at the time a case is identified. The concept of "risk set" is illustrated in Figure 1.

Risk set 1

	W28	W29	Risk set 1 W30	W31	W32	Risk set 2 W33	W34	W35	Risk set 3 W36	W37	W38	W39	W40
A	0	0	0	0	0	X							
B	0	0	0	0	0	0	0	0	0	0	0	0	0
C	0	0	X										
D	0	0	0	0	0	0	0	0	0	0	0	0	0
E	0	0	0	0	0	0	0	0	X				
F	0	0	0	0	0	0	0	0	0	0	0	0	0
G	0	0	0	0	0	0	0	0	0	0	0	0	0
H	0	0	0	0	0	0	0	0	0	0	0	0	0

Stillbirth X	Ongoing Pregnancy 0

Figure 1. A Hypothetical Case Cohort Study of Stillbirth.

In this cohort of eight pregnancies (A–H) that were followed from week 28 to week 40, three cases of stillbirth occurred. During week 30, when the first stillbirth (C) occurred, all other pregnancies were undelivered. The risk set at week 30 comprised all eight pregnancies, of which pregnancy C was the case and all the rest served as controls. Note that pregnancies A and E, which later became cases, served as controls for case C. The risk set for the second stillbirth included only seven pregnancies, of which A became a case, while C was not included in the risk set, as at that time it was no longer at risk. Pregnancy E, however, was included in the risk set. At the time stillbirth E occurred, the risk set included only six pregnancies, of which E was the case and the other five pregnancies (B, D, F, G and H) served as controls. In a regular case-control study, only the latter five pregnancies would have served as controls.

This methodology has been used in perinatal epidemiology, as it allows for optimal utilization of exposure information. In a study investigating risk factors for stillbirth, cases were identified through perinatal databases in Nova Scotia and Eastern Ontario, Canada 1991–2001 [20]. Exposure information was measured retrospectively from a sample of cases and controls. To account for differing lengths of gestation at the time of stillbirth, survival analysis approach was used, comparing cases to a comparison group (risk set) which included an original control group and a random sample of pregnancies which became cases in a later gestational week.

CROSS-SECTIONAL STUDIES

In cross-sectional studies, exposure and outcomes are assessed at the same time. This study design provides a low level of evidence because the temporal direction cannot be determined. The cross-sectional approach is used in population surveys, which provide important information on prevalence of risk factors in sub groups of the population. This information enables the identification of populations at risk. Information obtained from large monitoring of ongoing surveys such as the National Health Interview Survey (NHIS) [21], Behavioral Risk Factor Surveillance System (BRFSS) [22], Pregnancy Risk Assessment Monitoring System (PRAMS) [23] in the US and the Peristat survey in Europe [24] serve as the basis for initiation and evaluation of significant public health interventions.

ECOLOGICAL STUDIES

Ecological studies are based on comparing disease occurrence or prevalence in units of populations (countries, neighborhoods, towns, geographic areas, etc.) that are characterized by some exposure that is hypothesized to affect the likelihood of disease. Unlike all other study designs discussed so far, in ecological studies we do not study individuals but units of population; thus, neither disease status nor exposure status are determined at the individual level. This type of study is used for generating hypotheses and to evaluate community interventions. An ecological study design was recently used to evaluate a national public health intervention in Brazil [25]. The findings from this study, which compared infant mortality rates in municipalities with varying degrees of exposure to the public health intervention, demonstrated an inverse association between infant mortality rates and level of coverage of the national intervention program.

COMPARING THE USE AND STRENGTH OF EVIDENCE OF DIFFERENT STUDY DESIGNS IN OBSERVATIONAL PERINATAL EPIDEMIOLOGY

Four major categories of observational study designs were described: cohort, case-control, cross-sectional and ecological studies. Cohort studies provide the strongest type of evidence, as it follows the natural process from exposure to disease occurrence. Cohort studies are especially useful in perinatal epidemiology, as follow-up time in many studies is relatively short. The main difficulty with cohort studies is that they might lengthy, if conducted prospectively , and costly if large number of persons are to be followed. Cohort studies, relative to other observational study designs, are less prone to biases, as exposure status is determined before disease status is known. The main threat to validity in cohort studies is selection bias, which may be caused by selective participation in the study and/or selective drop from follow-up.

Case-control studies require fewer resources, as they are conducted on relatively small samples and for short periods of time. They are particularly efficient in the study of rare outcomes, but are more prone to both selection and information bias. If properly conducted, they can provide a valid estimate of association between exposure and disease. In contrast to cohort and case-control studies, cross-sectional and ecological studies cannot provide etiological evidence, but are very useful in providing population-based data on the prevalence of a variety of exposures and clinical conditions, and as a basis for evaluating interventions and changes at the population level.

REFERENCES

[1]   Gardiner HM.Early environmental influences on vascular development. *Early Hum Dev*. 2007 Dec;83(12):819-23.

[2]   Kajantie E. Fetal origins of stress-related adult disease. *Ann N Y Acad Sci*. 2006 Nov;1083:11-27.

[3]   Riboli E, Kaaks R. The EPIC Project: rationale and study design. European Prospective Investigation into Cancer and Nutrition. *Int J Epidemiol*. 1997;26 Suppl 1:S6-14.

[4]   Zetterström K, Lindeberg SN, Haglund B, Hanson U. The association of maternal chronic hypertension with perinatal death in male and female offspring: a record linkage study of 866,188 women. *BJOG*. 2008 Oct;115(11):1436-42.

[5]   Chen X, Scholl TO. Association of elevated free fatty acids during late pregnancy with preterm delivery. *Obstet Gynecol*. 2008 Aug;112(2 Pt 1):297-303.

[6]   Wisborg K, Barklin A, Hedegaard M, Henriksen TB Psychological stress during pregnancy and stillbirth: prospective study. *BJOG*. 2008 Jun;115(7):882-5.

[7]   Ness RB, Soper DE, Richter HE, Randall H, Peipert JF, Nelson DB, Schubeck D, McNeeley SG, Trout W, Bass DC, Hutchison K, Kip K, Brunham RC. Chlamydia antibodies, chlamydia heat shock protein, and adverse sequelae after pelvic inflammatory disease: the PID Evaluation and Clinical Health (PEACH). *Study. Sex Transm Dis*. 2008 Feb;35(2):129-35.

[8]   Jaddoe VW, van Duijn CM, van der Heijden AJ, Mackenbach JP, Moll HA, Steegers EA, Tiemeier H, Uitterlinden AG, Verhulst FC, Hofman A. The Generation R Study: design and cohort update until the age of 4 years. *Eur J Epidemiol*. 2008 Dec 20.

[9]   Friedlander Y, Paltiel O, Deutsch L, Knaanie A, Massalha S, Tiram E, Harlap S. Birthweight and relationship with infant, child and adult mortality in the Jerusalem perinatal study. *Paediatr Perinat Epidemiol*. 2003 Oct;17(4):398-406.

[10]   Johnson KJ, Spector LG, Klebanoff MA, Ross JA. Childhood cancer and birthmarks in the Collaborative Perinatal Project. *Pediatrics*. 2007 May;119(5):e1088-93.

[11] Cheng YW, Chung JH, Kurbisch-Block I, Inturrisi M, Shafer S, Caughey AB. Gestational weight gain and gestational diabetes mellitus: perinatal outcomes. *Obstet Gynecol.* 2008 Nov;112(5):1015-22.

[12] Ben-Joseph R, Levy A, Wiznitzer A, Holcberg G, Mazor M, Sheiner E. Pregnancy outcome of patients following deep venous thrombosis. *Matern Fetal Neonatal Med.* 2008 Dec 16:1-5.

[13] Ofir D, Levy A, Wiznitzer A, Mazor M, Sheiner E. Familial Mediterranean fever during pregnancy: An independent risk factor for preterm delivery. *Eur J Obstet Gynecol Reprod Biol.* 2008 Dec;141(2):115-8.

[14] Lundgren EM, Cnattingius S, Jonsson B, Tuvemo T. Birth characteristics and different dimensions of intellectual performance in young males: a nationwide population-based study. *Acta Paediatr.* 2003 Oct;92(10):1138-43.

[15] Philibert M, Deneux-Tharaux C, Bouvier-Colle MH. Can excess maternal mortality among women of foreign nationality be explained by suboptimal obstetric care? *BJOG.* 2008 Oct;115(11):1411-8.

[16] Vogt G, Puhó E, Czeizel AE. Population-based case-control study of isolated congenital cataract. *Birth Defects Res A Clin Mol Teratol.* 2005 Dec;73(12):997-1005.

[17] Kanagalingam MG, Nelson SM, Freeman DJ, Ferrell WR, Cherry L, Lowe GD, Greer IA, Sattar N. Vascular dysfunction and alteration of novel and classic cardiovascular risk factors in mothers of growth restricted offspring. *Atherosclerosis.* 2008 Oct 14.

[18] Szklow M. & Nieto FJ. (2007) *Epidemiology Beyond the Basics*, 2nd Edition. Sudbury MA, Jones and Bartlett Publishers.

[19] Bluhm E, McNeil DE, Cnattingius S, Gridley G, El Ghormli L, Fraumeni JF Jr. Int J Cancer. 2008 Dec 15;123(12):2885-90. Prenatal and perinatal risk factors for neuroblastoma. *Int J Cancer.* 2008 Dec 15;123(12):2885-90.

[20] Dodds L, King WD, Fell DB, Armson BA, Allen A, Nimrod C. Stillbirth risk factors according to timing of exposure. *Ann Epidemiol.* 2006 Aug;16(8):607-13.

[21] *www.cdc.gov/nchs/nhis*

[22] *http://www.cdc.gov/BRFSS/*

[23] *http://www.cdc.gov/prams/*

[24] *http://www.europeristat.com/*

[25] Aquino R, de Oliveira NF, Barreto ML. Impact of the family health program on infant mortality in Brazilian municipalities. *Am J Public Health.* 2009 Jan;99(1):87-93

In: Handbook of Methodological Concepts in Perinatal Medicine   ISBN: 978-1-62081-252-5
Editor: Eyal Sheiner   © 2013 Nova Science Publishers, Inc.

Chapter 4

RANDOMIZED, DOUBLE-BLIND, PLACEBO CONTROLLED TRIALS: ARE THEY REALLY THE "GOLD" STANDARD?

Anthony Odibo[*]

Women's and Fetal Imaging, Division of Ultrasound and Genetics,
Fetal Care Center, Department of Obstetrics and Gynecology,
Washington University School of Medicine,
St Louis, MO, US

DEFINITIONS

- Randomized controlled trials (RCT): Studies investigating efficacy or effectiveness of treatment, involving random allocation of different interventions (treatments or conditions) to patients, ensuring that known and unknown confounders are evenly distributed between treatment groups.
- Double-blind trial: The researcher and the patients do not know whether the treatment is a drug rather a placebo (or new vs. old drug). Double-blind trials tend to give accurate results since the researcher cannot possibly consult the patient, directly or otherwise, and cannot give in to patient pressure to give him the new treatment.

INTRODUCTION

Clinical research, including those in perinatology, attempt to mimic the laboratory model of research design by employing rigorous methods to reduce the introduction of bias and confounding into the final outcome. The randomized, double-blind placebo-controlled design has come to be regarded as the "gold-standard" to which other designs of clinical research

[*] Correspondence: Anthony Odibo, MD, MSCE, Division of Maternal Fetal Medicine, Department of Obstetrics and Gynecology., Washington University in St Louis, 4990 Children's Place, St Louis MO, 63110, odiboa@wudosis.wustl.edu.

should be compared. [1] This chapter highlights the advantages of the randomized controlled trial (RCT) compared with other study designs, but also sounds a note of caution in the conduct and interpretation of the results of these trials and begs the question that they may not always represent the "gold-standard".

AN OVERVIEW OF RANDOMIZED-CONTROLLED TRIALS

When properly conducted, a RCT provide the most reliable basis for evaluating the efficacy and safety of new treatments. They provide the most convincing demonstration of causality. The main reason for randomization is to avoid bias due to imbalance of known and unknown confounders between the groups being studied. [2] Typical examples of study designs using the RCT approach include: comparing a new drug vs placebo; new combinations of drugs vs single drug; new surgical procedure or device.

A detailed discussion of RCT is beyond the scope of this chapter, however, a brief description of the process will be provided as a backdrop for the limitations to be highlighted later on.

In designing a RCT, the primary end point is crucial. The end-point must be well-defined, reproducible, clinically relevant and easily achievable. [2] The sample size consideration for the study is usually driven by the chosen end-point. Typical end-points can be continuous or ordinal data, may involve the use of rates of events or time-to event considerations. When the primary clinical outcome may involve a very long period to conduct or if very expensive, it is not uncommon to use surrogate markers that may provide quicker results.

When using surrogate markers certain principles must be considered. An ideal surrogate marker should be reproducible, easily measured, occur at a stage that is earlier than the main clinical outcome of interest, and of course related to the clinical outcome. The surrogate outcome should be amenable to treatment in trials involving therapy. Examples of surrogate markers or end-points include: the use of CD4 counts or viral load as indicators of response to HIV therapy, low density lipoproteins (LDL) as surrogates for cardiac events in studies involving heart disease or tumor size as a measure of response to chemotherapy.

There are other important practical issues that need to be addressed at the planning phase of a RCT. These include choosing the proper control groups; deciding on the method of randomization such as the use of coin flip, random table numbers or computer generated random numbers; the appropriateness of blinding and method of blinding including placebo or sham surgery; the number of study arms which is most commonly a two-arm study, but some may employ a cross-over design using an appropriate wash-out period. Finally, the study planning committee needs to decide what they actually want to accomplish with the study. Do they want to prove that a new therapy is superior or equally efficient compared with an established therapy? The sample size consideration can be influenced by such decisions of equivalence/non-inferiority versus superiority designs. [2]

Table 1. The strengths and weaknesses of randomized controlled trials

Strengths	Weaknesses
Best design for evaluating causal relationship	Ethical issues with randomization
Can control bias	Expensive to conduct
Can measure multiple outcomes	Issues with compliance

The overall strengths of RCT is that they are the best design for evaluating a causal relationship in a study and for controlling bias and that they can be used to measure multiple outcomes. The RCT design however can be expensive, may encounter certain ethical hurdles that make their conduct difficult and there may be issues with compliance depending on the group to which subjects are randomized and whether their underlying medical condition is apparently improving or worsening. The strengths and weakness of RCT are depicted in Table 1. There are certain biases that can result from poor conduction of RCT including detection or classification bias, co-interventions and contaminations. This chapter will assume that the RCT is well conducted but highlight the possible systematic errors that could occur in an ideal RCT.

THE DISCREPANCY DEBATE

The implied objectivity of a double-blind RCT is the differential outcomes that it can detect when compared with other research designs. [3] It had always been assumed that other study designs tend to overestimate treatment effects when compared with the RCT. [4] This discrepancy in treatment effects between RCTs and other research designs has been termed the "masking bias" and is generally accepted as evidence of the objectivity of blinded RCTs. [5]

In the report of the first study that introduced the term "double-blind" to clinicians, Gold and colleagues also introduced the "discrepancy debate" using the pilot study of the cardiac drug Khellin. [6,7] The pilot study of Khellin involved 19 patients and demonstrated dramatic improvement in cardiac indices compared with placebo. A larger double-blind study involving 39 patients showed no benefit in the use of the cardiac drug compared with placebo. [7] In short, most of the early studies establishing the objectivity of RCT proved that the more rigorous and stringent the methodology, the less efficacious the therapy and reinforced the belief that less rigorous methods produced higher estimates in favor of therapy. [8-13]

However, recently conducted systematic reviews of study designs have compounded the discrepancy debate in that they confirm that poor methodology in other study designs could bias results but in either direction of over-estimating or under-estimating the treatment effect when compared with RCT. [14-17] These systematic reviews resulted in a modified proposition of the discrepancy argument and Kuntz and Oxman now propose the RCT as the "best protection against the unpredictability of bias". [14]

Can the Process of RCT Result in Significant Bias?

In clinical research, we are dealing with conscious beings and some form of uncertainty could cloud even the most rigorous scientific process. The proponents of the discrepancy debate assume that deficiencies such as selection and measurement bias are responsible for the differences seen between RCT and other research designs. However, even the ideal experimental conditions can have unpredictable influence on clinical outcomes.

The set up for most RCTs are not the same as those in regular clinical settings and this can on its own result in biased results. [18,19] The participants in RCTs can also exhibit similar unconscious responses that distort the results as we see with other study designs. The knowledge that the subjects have a chance of receiving either a placebo or the actual therapy introduces uncertain perceptions in the patient enough to decrease the response of either the placebo or the medication.

The preferences of the patients are taken away by the RCT process and could result in confusion, demoralization and even poor compliance, all of which may influence the study results. These have been termed "resentful demoralization" and "voluntary submission" by certain authors. [20, 21] There is also the potential that post-randomization processes such as increased vigilance may result in increased drug effect or decreased placebo effect or vice versa. [22] Some of these factors may distort the underlying statistical assumption that the "placebo effect" in the treatment arm is similar to that in the placebo arm. [23]

The Possibility of a "Masking Bias" in Rcts

The ideal method of testing the "gold-standard" and verify the validity of the masked RCT study is to design a study where both the patients and the dispensing physicians are unaware that they are involved in a blind RCT. This has been termed the "platinum standard" by Kaptchuk. [3] Such a study may however, be impossible due to ethical barriers. As an alternative certain studies using some form of "deception" to evaluate the possibility of masking bias have been performed. [6, 24]

In one study, 30 matched hospitalized patients with insomnia were randomized to a double-blind RCT. One group of patients were informed they were in a RCT comparing place to a hypnotic drug ("benzodiazepine") while the other matched group were not informed of being in a study. Eventually, both groups received a single dose of a placebo. The control group that were unaware of being in a study reported a higher hypnotic effect compared with the first group. [24] In another study involving cancer patients receiving naproxen versus placebo, who were randomly chosen to be informed of being in a RCT or not, the "placebo" was significantly more effective in the informed group than naproxen in the uninformed group! [25] These two studies were performed in France before informed consent became mandatory.

Although the result of the insomnia and the pain studies above were opposite, the second study proved that awareness of being in a masked RCT compared with uninformed involvement in RCT produce disproportionate effects on the placebo and active drug. This would also suggest that a significant difference in the placebo response of the treatment arm versus the placebo arm unlike the traditional statistical assumption.

There are many other examples in the literature that confirm that for many active drugs that can be distinguished by the subject if they know what to expect, complete concealment can dramatically change the pharmacological effects. [26-29]

It must be emphasized that these effects of "deception" or concealments described above mainly concern short term effects and may not apply to RCTs evaluating long-term outcomes. [3]

Other Sources of Bias in RCTs

While patients are randomized in RCTs, in most cases, the investigators are not. It is a known fact that most researchers are different from the typical clinician and studies have shown that different researchers have different abilities to elicit placebo effect on subjects. [18] In one study, it was shown that with the same placebo, two different researchers either consistently increased or consistently decreased patient's gastric secretion! [30] The above has been described as "investigator self-selection" bias. Different styles of health care provision can result in measurable differences in outcomes and such effects have been confirmed in studies where the physician was made an independent variable. [31, 32] One suggestion for addressing this effect is to have a "physician run-in phase in RCTs to eliminate the influence of practitioners on the integrity of RCTs. [33]

The psychosocial literature have several examples that demonstrate that the process of negotiating therapy between patients and their physicians affects not only compliance but also hard outcomes such as survival. [34, 35] The process of randomization in RCTs removes such patients' preferences and could introduce a type of "preference bias". Such influences are more typical in studies involving un-blinded studies involving behavioral changes such as dieting and exercise. [36]

Table 2. Potential factors resulting in bias in a well conducted randomized controlled trial

Experimental conditions of RCT are not similar to typical clinical scenarios
Patients preference and "resentful demoralization"
Post-randomization influences on the "placebo effect"
Investigator "self-selection" bias
"Consent" versus "non-consenting" bias: subjects in RCT are atypical patients

Other human influences can creep in and influence the outcomes of RCTs. It is common knowledge that the typical patient that consent to participate in a RCT, is usually different from the average patient. Many eligible subjects may decline participation and his can potentially bias the trial results. One study showed that the typical patients that consent to studies involving therapy are less affluent and less educated while the opposite is the case for typical consenters to prevention trials. [37] Such "consent" or "non-consent" bias may result in different outcomes in RCT when compared with typical clinical scenarios. The above examples of bias in RCTs are highlighted in Table 2.

Examples from Perinatal Literature

Due to practical and ethical difficulties with blinding during pregnancy, some of the examples above are not easily demonstrated in the perinatal literature. There are however, some indirect, but unproven evidence that can be examined.

The trial by Meis et al on behalf of the MFMU network, concluded that 17-hydroxy progesterone can prevent preterm birth in the treatment group. While it does not detract from the positive effect of therapy in the treatment group, the preterm delivery rate of 54.5% in the control group was much higher than would be expected. [38] The unanswered question is whether the placebo had additional detrimental effect in addition to the prior history of preterm birth in both groups.

Another consideration from the perinatal literature is in regard to studies comparing treatments for prevention of preterm birth such as cerclage to bed rest. [39,40] The assumption is that bed rest is not an intervention and therefore is comparable to a placebo. However, there are no trials out there comparing bed rest to routine activities for prevention of preterm birth that we are aware of. This may really be an example of poor choice of a control group rather than an inherent bias in RCT.

CONCLUSION

This chapter has highlighted the limitations of RCT, but it must be emphasized that RCTs are still the closest approximation to laboratory experiments. It has been demonstrated that blinded and un-blinded RCTs can introduce inherent sources of bias. The main aim of this chapter is to bring the attention of researchers to these potential sources of bias in the conduct and interpretation of RCTs. A secondary aim is to propose that when a well designed RCT is impossible, findings from properly conducted cohort studies should not be underestimated.

REFERENCES

[1]   Hennekens CH, Buring JE, Hebert PR. Implications of overviews of randomized trials. *Stat Med.* 1987;6(3):397-409.

[2]   Rothman KJ, Greenland S: Matching. In Rothman KJ, Greenland S. Modern Epidemiology, 2nd edition. Philadelphia: *Lippincott Williams and Williams*; p147-161.

[3]   Kaptchuk TJ. The double-blind, randomized, placebo-controlled trial: Gold standard or golden calf? *J Clin Epid* 2001; 54: 541-549.

[4]   Sibbald B, Roland M. Why are randomized controlled trials important?. *Br Med J.* 1998; 316:201–202.

[5]   Schulz KF, Chalmers I, Hayes RJ and D.G. Altman, Empirical evidence of bias. Dimensions of methodological quality associated with estimates of treatment effects in controlled trials. *J Am Med Assoc.* 1995; 273: 408–412.

[6]   Kaptchuk TJ. Intentional ignorance: a history of blind assessment and placebo controls. *Bull Hist Med.* 1998; 72:389–433.

[7]   Greiner T, Gold H, Cattell M, Travell J, Bakst H, Rinzler SH, Benjamin ZH, Warshaw LJ, Bobb AL, Kwit NT, Modell W, Rothendler HH, Messeloff CR, Kramer ML. A method for the evaluation of the effects of drugs on cardiac pain in patients with angina on effort. A study of Khellin (Visammin). *Am J Med.* 1950; 9:143–155.

[8]   Foulds GA. Clinical research in psychiatry. *J Ment Sci.*1958; 104:259–265.

[9]   Glick BS, Margolis R. A study of the influence of experimental design on clinical outcome in drug research. *Am J Psychol.* 1962; 118:1087–1096.

[10]   Astin A, Ross S, Glutamic acid and human intelligence. *Psychol Bull.* 1960; 57: 429–434.

[11]   Wechsler H, Grosser GH, Greenblatt M. Research evaluating antidepressant medications on hospitalized mental patients: a survey of published reports during a five-year period. *J Nerve Ment Dis.* 1965; 141:231–239.

[12]   Grace ND, Muench H, Chalmer TC. The present status of shunts for portal hypertension in cirrhosis. *Gastroenterology.* 1996; 50: 684–691.

[13]   O'Brien WM. Indomethacin: a survey of clinical trials. *Clin Pharm Ther.* 1967; 9: 94–107.

[14]   Kunz R, Oxman AD. The unpredictability paradox: review of empirical comparisons of randomized and non-randomized clinical trials. *Br Med J.* 1998; 317:1185–1190.

[15]   Recurrent Miscarriage Immunotherapy Trialists Group. Worldwide collaborative observational study and meta-analysis on allogenic leukocyte immunotherapy for recurrent spontaneous abortion. *Am J Reprod Immunol.* 1994; 32:55–72.

[16]   Miller JN, Colditz GA, Mosteller F. How study design affects outcomes in comparisons of therapy. II: surgical. *Stat Med.* 1989; 8:455–466.

[17]   Ottenbacher K. Impact of random assignment on study outcome: an empirical examination. *Control Clin Trials.* 1992;13:50–61.

[18]   Black N. Why we need observational studies to evaluate the effectiveness of health care. *Br Med J.* 1996; 312:1215–1218.

[19]   McPherson K. The best and the enemy of the good: randomised controlled trials, uncertainty, and assessing the role of patient choice in medical decision making. *J Epidemiol Comm Health.* 1994; 48: 6–15.

[20]   Torgerson DJ, Sibbald B. What is a patient preference trial? *Br Med J.* 1998; 316: 360.

[21]   Silverman WA, Altman DG. Patients' preferences and randomized trials. *Lancet.* 1996; 347:171–174.

[22]   Kempthorne O. Why randomize? *J Stat Plan Inf.* 1977; 1:1–25.

[23]   Kaptchuk TJ. Powerful placebo: the dark side of the randomized controlled trial. *Lancet.*1998; 351:1722–1725.

[24]   Dahan R, Caulin C, Figea L, Kanis JA, Cauline R, Segrestaa JM. Does informed consent influence therapeutic outcome? A clinical trial of the hypnotic activity of placebo in patients admitted to hospital. *Br Med J.* 1986; 293:363–364.

[25]   Bergmann JF, Chassany O, Gandiol J, Deblois P, Kanis JA, Segrestaa JM, Caulin C, Dahan R. A randomized clinical trial of the effect of informed consent on the analgesic activity of placebo and naproxen in cancer pain. *Clin Trials Meta-Anal.* 1994; 29: 41–47.

[26]   Kirsch I, Weixel LJ. Double-blind versus deceptive administration of a placebo. *Behav Neurosci.* 1988; 2:319–323.

[27] Hughes JR, Gulliver SB, Amori G, Mireault GC, Fenwsick JF. Effect of instructions and nicotine on smoking cessation, withdrawal symptoms and self-administration of nicotine gum. *Psychopharmacology.* 1989;99:486–491.

[28] Kirsch I, Rosadino MJ. Do double-blind studies with informed consent yield externally valid results?. *Psychopharmacology.* 1993;110:437–442.

[29] Dinnerstein AJ, Lowenthal M, Blitz B. The interaction of drugs with placebos in the control of pain and anxiety. *Perspect Biol Med.* 1966;10:103–114.

[30] Wolf S. Part IV. Placebos: problems and pitfalls. *Clin Pharmacol Ther.* 1962; 3: 254–257.

[31] LeBaron S, Reyher J, Stack JM. Paternalistic vs. egalitarian physician styles: the treatment of patients in crisis. *J Fam Med.* 1985; 21:56–62.

[32] Sarles H, Camatte R, Sahel J. A study of the variations in the response regarding duodenal ulcer when treated with placebo by different investigators. *Digestion.* 1977;16:289–292.

[33] Shapiro AK, Shapiro E. The powerful placebo: from ancient priest to modern physician, *The Johns Hopkins University Press,* Baltimore (1997).

[34] Horwitz RI, Viscolli CM, Berkman L, Donaldson RM, Horwitz SM, Murray CJ, Ransohoff DF, Sindelar J. Treatment adherence and risk of death after a myocardial infarction. *Lancet.* 1991; 336:543–545.

[35] Horwitz RI, Horwitz SM. Adherence to treatment and health outcomes. *Arch Intern Med.* 1993; 153:1863–1868.

[36] Brewin CR, Bradley C. Patient preferences and randomised clinical trials. *Br Med J.* 1989; 299: 313–315.

[37] McKee M, Gritton A, Black N, McPherson K, Sanderson C, Bain C. Interpreting the evidence: choosing between randomized and non-randomized studies. *Br Med J.*1999; 319:312–315.

[38] Meis PJ, Klebanoff M, Thom E, Dombrowski MP, Sibai B, Moawad AH, Spong CY, Hauth JC, Miodovnik M, Varner MW, Leveno KJ, Caritis SN, Iams JD, Wapner RJ, Conway D, O'Sullivan MJ, Carpenter M, Mercer B, Ramin SM, Thorp JM, Peaceman AM, Gabbe S; National Institute of Child Health and Human Development Maternal-Fetal Medicine Units Network. Prevention of recurrent preterm delivery by 17 alpha-hydroxyprogesterone caproate. *N Engl J Med.* 2003;349(13): 1299.

[39] Berghella V, Odibo AO, Tolosa JE.. Cerclage for prevention of preterm birth in women with a short cervix found on transvaginal ultrasound examination: a randomized trial. *Am J Obstet Gynecol.* 2004; 191(4):1311-7.

[40] Berghella V, Odibo AO, To MS, Rust OA, Althuisius SM. Cerclage for short cervix on ultrasonography: meta-analysis of trials using individual patient-level data. *Obstet Gynecol.* 2005;106(1):181-9.

In: Handbook of Methodological Concepts in Perinatal Medicine   ISBN: 978-1-62081-252-5
Editor: Eyal Sheiner   © 2013 Nova Science Publishers, Inc.

Chapter 5

DATA ANALYSIS

Julia Harris and Eyal Sheiner[*]

Department of Obstetrics and Gynecology, Soroka University Medical Center and the
Faculty of Health Sciences, Ben-Gurion University of the Negev, Beer-Sheva, Israel

INTRODUCTION

The use of clear and appropriate statistics in medical research is crucial for the generation of useful outcomes that can benefit the medical community. In order to produce such statistics, it is necessary to master the basic principles of biostatistics. Firstly, one must be comfortable with the terminology and tools that comprise basic biostatistics. [1]

VARIABLES

Variables, or measurable characteristics of a sample population, are categorized so that diverse data can be easily compared and understood by those who did not conduct the research. Furthermore, these categorizations determine what type of statistics can be garnered from the data since the categorizations are based on intrinsic characteristics of the data set. For example, one way to describe a variable is by whether it is continuous or not. A continuous variable has numerical values that exist on an uninterrupted ordinal scale. An example is birth weight (figure 1) [2], or cervical length (figure 2) [3]. It is important to note that continuous variables are measured on a scale with comparable intervals. For example, a baby of 2.0 kilograms is exactly one half the weight of a baby weighing 4.0 kilograms.

Variables that are not continuous are considered discrete; the values of discrete variables are often referred to as ordinal or categorical. A discrete variable has values that are non-numerical and are not comparable as their intervals are not equivalent. Discrete variables can be further categorized by their number of outcomes. For example, sex is a dichotomous

[*] Corresponding author: Eyal Sheiner, M.D, PhD, Department of Obstetrics and Gynecology, Soroka University Medical Center, P.O Box 151, Faculty of Health Science, Ben-Gurion University of the Negev, Beer-Sheva, Israel., Tel 972-8-6403551 Fax 972-8-6403294, E-mail: sheiner@bgu.ac.il.

discrete variable; this is a non-numerical variable with two possible outcomes. Variables can also be categorized as quantitative or qualitative variables based on whether their outcome characteristic is measurable such as the number of births, a quantitative variable or a characteristic with no ordering or numerical value attached to its outcome such as religion, a qualitative variable.

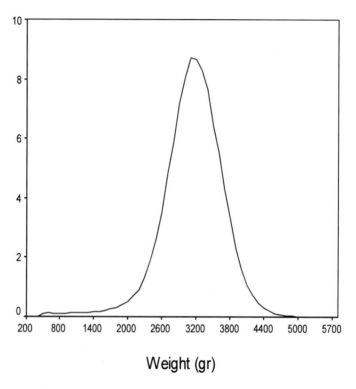

Weight (gr)

Figure 1. Birth weight distribution of 199,093 deliveries in the Soroka University Medical Center, Beer-Sheva, Israel during the years 1988-2007. [2]

A complex application of the multiple ways to categorize variables discussed above can be found in a study titled *Gender Does Matter in Perinatal Medicine*, [4] where sex is used as a discrete, qualitative, dichotomous variable. This article found that the sex of a fetus (i.e. male vs. female) can be used as an indicator for increased risk of perinatal complications such as gestational diabetes mellitus, fetal macrosomia and failure to progress during the first and second stages of labor.

DESCRIPTIVE STATISTICS

Once variables have been defined and measured, the next step is to draw conclusions from the data collected. Firstly, one must should describe the data using what is called descriptive statistics. These statistics serve to summarize the basic features of the sample population from which the data wereas obtained. Which descriptive statistics best portray the sample are determined by the types of variables collected. If the study involves continuous variables, the most important and most commonly used descriptive statistics are the mean, median and mode.

$$\bar{x} = \frac{1}{n}\sum_{i=1}^{n} x_i = \frac{1}{n}(x_1 + \cdots + x_n).$$

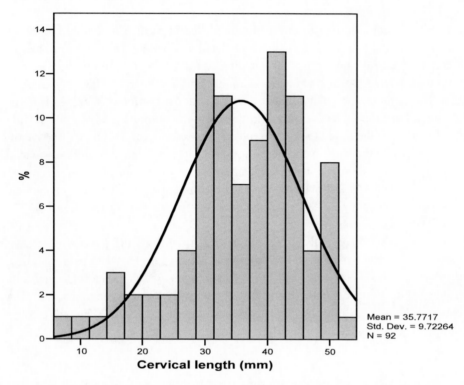

Figure 2. Cervical length in millimeters, measured by ultrasound, among 92 women with idiopathic polyhydramnios. [3]

$$\bar{x} = \frac{1}{n}\sum_{i=1}^{n} x_i = \frac{1}{n}(x_1 + \cdots + x_n).$$

The mean is calculated as follows (see above): one divides the summation of the values of a given variable by n (the number of participants) for which said variable was collected. This statistic is used to express the "average," or the most reflective value for a given population. Another statistic commonly employed as a representative value for a given sample population is the median. This statistic is the value which divides the data set into two; half of the values for the variable lie above the median and half lie below. If n is an even number, to obtain the median one must calculate the mean of the two values which saddle the centermost data point; the greatest value of the lower half of the data set and the least value of the upper half of the data set. Thirdly, there is a statistic called the mode. The mode is the most frequently found value for a given variable.

The best way to demonstrate the use of descriptive statistics is to observe their direct application in research. Figure 3 represents the thermal index for bones (TIB) measured during B-mode ultrasound studies. [5] TIB expresses the potential for rise in temperature at the ultrasound's focal point. In this TIB data set, the mean and mode were similar (i.e. 0.3). When a data set yields such results, called a *unimodal* distribution, the mode can be very useful. A unimodal distribution is a data set that contains a highly concentrated set of values for a single variable (figures 1, 2 and 4).

Another useful descriptive statistic commonly used in medical research is a proportion. This statistic is similar to a percentage. It is calculated by dividing the number of observations with a certain characteristic by n, thus yielding the percentage or proportion of the total observations that have the characteristic in mind. This measure can be very useful when dealing with a variable with integral values, such as the proportion of fatalities from uterine cancer in which metastases had occurred. In this case, the proportion would be equivalent to what is referred to as the case-fatality rate (of uterine cancer), or the number of fatalities per number of cases with the same pathology. Proportions can also be used to draw conclusions and compare data. For example, one can determine if a proportion of a specific population that contracts an illness is larger than average (by comparison to a national or international statistic) or larger than would be expected to occur by chance. These concepts will be elaborated below.

When using descriptive statistics to summarize a data set, the goal is either to show similarity within a data set or to show difference, which is referred to as variability. The mean, median and mode represent similarity of data points within a data set, which can also be referred to as measures of central tendency. Alternatively, some common ways in which to represent statistical variability include: standard deviation (SD), standard error (SE), interquartile range, range, variance and the coefficient of variation.

MEASURES OF STATISTICAL VARIABILITY

Standard deviation (SD) is the average distance that values fall from the mean. SD is calculated by summing the squared distances from the mean, dividing this sum by n or by $n - 1$ and taking the square root of the entire value. The value of $n-1$ is often used as the SD denominator because it accounts for a loss in the degrees of freedom, the number of observations that are free to vary. Every time that a calculation is done, a degree of freedom is lost in the manipulation of the data set and therefore needs to be taken into account by subtracting one from the value of n, yielding a more accurate statistic. Within samples that are normally distributed (figures 1 and 4), 68.0% of the sample will fall within one SD, 95.0% of the sample population will fall within 1.96 SDs, and 95.4% will fall within two SDs. The intervals of values that fall within the bounds of SDs can also be called confidence intervals (CIs) and are used to describe the population from which the sample is drawn.

Confidence intervals are used to make statements about normally distributed variables, such as the following: with a 95% CI, it can be assumed that the mean birth weight of a population is between 3510 and 4490 grams. In this example, the mean birth weight of the sample (note: a sample is a slice taken from a larger population in the hopes of obtaining data reflective of the population which cannot be studied in its entirety) was 4000g, with an SD of

250g. Therefore, there is a 95% chance that the mean birth weight of this population should fall within the stated range of values: 3510g - 4490g, based on the idea that statistically we know that 95% of the sampled participants' birth weights can be found within two SDs. This value is calculated as follows, the SD, 250g, is multiplied by 1.96 in order to give a 95% CI of 490g which is applied to either side of the mean, giving the range 3510g - 4490g. This range has a 95% chance of containing the mean birth weight of the population from which this sample was drawn.

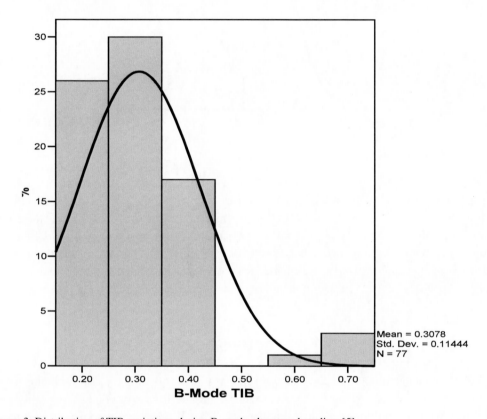

Figure 3. Distribution of TIB variations during B-mode ultrasound studies. [5]

Another value of interest, used in many statistical formulas is the variance (v). This value is obtained by squaring the SD. Variance therefore increases on an exponential scale whereas SD only increases incrementally; hence variance can be used to emphasize the variability within a data set. When the SD is divided by the square root of n, the resulting number is the standard error (SE) of the population. SE is used in many statistical tests; it can be viewed as the amount of variation contributed by each participant (see statistical tests section below for examples).

Interquartile range, another descriptive statistic of interest, is based on quartiles which are the subsections of the data set that result when it is divided into four equal sections called the first, second, third and fourth quartiles. The distance between the first and third quartiles is called the interquartile range, another measure of statistical dispersion. Range, which is incorporated into the interquartile range, is the distance between the smallest and largest values of a given data subset. The last descriptive statistic of interest is the coefficient of variation, which is the ratio of the SD to the mean.

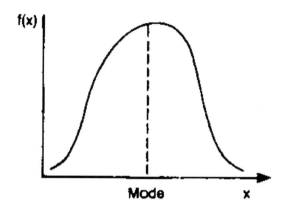

Figure 4. Normal distribution curve.

It is important to remember that variation in a clinical study can reflect one of two concepts: errors in data/data collection, or true variation within the population. It is not easy to differentiate these two types of variation without collecting more data from the same sample population. Simply keep in mind that variation in data, just as any observation one draws from a data set, may or may not be reflective of true characteristics of the population. Repetition of results has always been heralded in all sectors of science due to the fact that results obtained can always be due to the unforeseen interference of associated factors.

ERRORS

Errors in data are important and can also serve as tools for the interpretation of data. Type I errors, also known as false-positives occur when a certain disease or condition is said to be found in a patient who does not have this malady. Type II errors, commonly referred to as false-negatives, occur when a patient is not diagnosed with an illness which he or she possesses (Table 1).

By manipulating the values defined above one can generate multiple other useful statistics, see Table 1 and its subscript. One such value is the sensitivity, which can be defined as the percent of patients who have the disease that are correctly identified, or the true positives/(true positives + false negatives). A useful way of evaluating the efficacy of a diagnostic test is to compare, the sensitivity of an exam to the number of false-negative diagnoses. When this ratio is made (sensitivity of a test/ false negative error rate) a new value is obtained called the likelihood ratio (LR). An LR involving the false-positive error rate also exists and is referred to as the LR+ or the positive likelihood ratio. When a diagnostic test yields an LR greater than 1, it is considered a valid exam.

When the LR- is graphed, the result is called a receiver operating characteristic curve (ROC; figure 5 [6]). This curve can be used to identify an appropriate cut-off point for a diagnostic exam or to draw other conclusions that can be obtained from the relationship between sensitivity (true-positive rate) and the false-positive rate. For example, ROC analysis was employed to investigate the ability of birth weight to predict shoulder dystocia. [6,7].This study included the area under the curve (AUC) of the ROC due to its high predictive value of birth weight: AUC 0.92, 95% CI 0.90-0.93; p<0.001. [6,7].

Table 1. Comparing the results of a test with the actual disease status

	Disease	No Disease
Positive Test	True Positive (TP)	False Positive (FP)
Negative Test	False Negative (FN)	True Negative (TN)

Sensitivity= TP/(TP+FN); Specificity=TN/(TN+FP).

In order to generate an ROC that is useful in predicting appropriate cut-off points, one must graph a variety of false-positive error rates from numerous studies against the sensitivity of these exams. The point closest to the top left corner of the graph will be the most accurate cut-off point because it has the highest sensitivity and the lowest false-positive error rate of the data graphed. By employing such a cut-off point, one is choosing a limited data range with a high probability of including accurately diagnosed subjects.

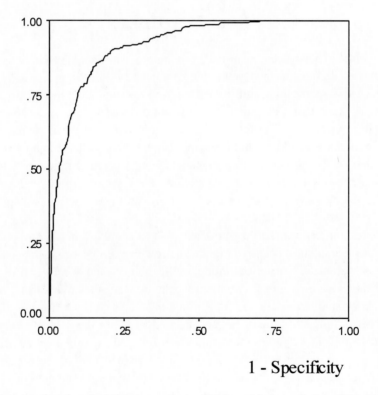

1 - Specificity

Figure 5. A receiver operating characteristic curve analysis of birth-weight in prediction of shoulder dystocia; based on analysis of 245 shoulder dystocia cases. [6]

DISTRIBUTIONS

All of the analyses thus far discussed operate on the assumption that the data are normally distributed (figure 4). When a given characteristic is measured in a population it is expected that the values obtained will congregate around a given number (the mean and/or median). Additionally, it is assumed that when plotted on a continuous scale, the experimental data will have a characteristic bell shaped curve surrounding this central value. This bell-shaped curve (figures 1 and 4), called the normal distribution has been found repeatedly in many studies and its presence allows for the efficacy of the various statistical tests and measures (of continuous variable) thus far mentioned. All statistical tests which rely on a normal distribution (or more rarely on another assumption about the data) are called parametric statistical tests.

Non-parametric statistical tests do not make such assumptions. These tests are useful for ranked data or data lacking numerical indices. For the purposes of perinatal epidemiology, only four of the most common and most relevant non-parametric tests will be discussed: the Kruskal-Wallis, the Mann-Whitney U or Wilcoxon rank sum test, chi-squared tests and Mantel-Haenszel.

NULL HYPOTHESIS

After variables have been identified, but before data is collected, it is customary to present a hypothesis, an educated prediction of outcomes. For the purposes of statistics, one must present two hypotheses, a null hypothesis and an alternative hypothesis. Commonly, a null hypothesis states that a statistically significant difference will not be found between the experimental group and the control group. The alternative hypothesis is that a difference of statistical significance will be found. Once the data has been collected and statistical tests are run that evaluate the presence of a statistically significant difference between the two experimental groups, the null hypothesis is either rejected or accepted. If the null hypothesis is rejected, the alternative hypothesis is not yet proven to be true, but rather is accepted as likely due to the statistical evidence.

Statistical significance is based on the idea that an event occurred more often in a sample population than would have occurred due to chance alone. Empirically, statistical significance is based upon parameters specified prior to collection of data. Firstly, an α value must be selected. This value represents the highest rate of false-positive errors that would be acceptable in the study to be conducted. A value of 0.05 is almost always used, which means that a type I error (a false-positive) can occur less than 5% of the time and the study will still be considered valid. This value is more commonly referred to as the p value of the study. It is stated that when p is less than 0.05, the result obtained can be considered statistically significant. If a researcher decides to employ the use of an α value greater than 0.05, he or she should justify the decision to do so, as most statistics only acknowledge significance when p is less than 0.05.

STATISTICAL TESTS

Once a *p* value has been identified, and data has been obtained, it is possible to perform statistical tests. The most commonly used tests in medical research are t-tests and z-tests. The t-test, also known as the Student's t-test, is employed when comparing the means of two groups (most often, a control group and an experimental group). These groups are selected from a normally distributed population for which the SD is unknown and therefore must be estimated from the data which ideally should have a small sample size (relative to the population). To summarize, the t-test compares the means of two groups that come from a small sample size taken from a normally distributed population for which the SD is unknown. The z-test, on the other hand, is used when comparing proportions instead of means, however; all of the conditions of the t-test apply.

Both the t-test and the z-test involve the calculation of a ratio called the critical ratio. This ratio compares the standard error (SE) to the statistical parameter being tested (i.e. either means or proportions depending upon the data). In the case of a t-test, the critical ratio is a comparison of the SE to the difference between two means. When working with z-tests, the critical ratio would involve the SE and the difference between two proportions. The two means or proportions involved in the calculation of the critical ratio should be chosen in such a way that they represent the control group and the experimental group respectively. Thus, if the control group and experimental group differ significantly, this will show in the critical ratio when the differences of their means or proportions are compared to the SE of the population. The following equation is used: Critical Ratio= difference between two means or proportions/SE of the difference between the two means or proportions.

NONPARAMETRIC TESTS

There are many other statistical tests which can be used. However, for the purposes of perinatal epidemiology the most relevant tests outside of t-tests and z-tests are Mann-Whitney U, Kruskal-Wallis, Chi-squared tests and the Mantel-Haensze, all of which can employ the use of nonparametric data. The Mantel-Haenszel test is also known as the Cochran-Mantel-Haenszel (CMH) test, it is used to compare two groups on a binary response.

Mann-Whitney U also called Mann-Whitney-Wilcoxon is similar to the Student's t-test in that it tests whether there is significant difference between two groups of data, most commonly the control and test groups. A null hypothesis is employed that states these data are similar enough that they could have been drawn from the same group. If the data are categorical, they need to be ranked and the mean ranks of each data set are compared to determine "difference" among them. If there is a large different difference between the ranks of these two data sets, the null hypothesis is rejected. Additionally, a t-test using the assigned ranks as if they were numerical observations can be done to ensure the significance of the Mann-Whitney result. In a recent study, aA Mann-Whitney test was used to determine if there was a significant difference in the Bishop scores of occiput posterior (OP) positioned births and non-OP positioned births. [8]. The study found there was no difference; therefore, according to the definition above, the null hypothesis was accepted.

A Kruskal-Wallis test is used to compare three or more groups of ordinal data (the version of this test that employs continuous data is called ANOVA). This test, like Mann-Whitney requires that ranks are assigned to the data. In Kruskal-Wallis the ranks of each data set are summed, and the means are calculated and compared to determine if the groups differ more than could be expected by chance. In one-way ANOVA, the same procedure is carried out with numerical, continuous data; this test usually employs the use of a statistical analysis program to ensure accuracy.

STATISTICAL MODELS

There are a variety of models created from mathematical equations that are used to explain data so that predictions can be made from the data and extended to the population at large. One such model incorporates the concept of null and alternative hypotheses, beginning with the statement that two variables are independent. If this statement can be sufficiently proven, the null hypothesis (no difference exists) is rejected and the alternative hypothesis is accepted. When utilizing this type of model, it is common to employ the use of a Chi-squared test ($\chi 2$). The Chi-square test is meant to prove the independence of two variables in a study. The model, in this case independence, provides an expected set of values. When one graphs the data values obtained in a study alongside those "expected" values based on a particular model, the chi-square test determines whether the data obtained fits sufficiently into the predicted model, it is a "goodness-of-fit" test. This test shows how far off the obtained values are from those values predicted using the chosen model. The outcomes measured in this case are referred to as "O" for obtained and "E" for expected values. Therefore the equation for chi-square is: $\chi 2 = \sum [\frac{(O-E)2}{E}]$. When a Chi-square value is small it means the outcomes are close to the expected, therefore the null hypothesis can be rejected and if $\chi 2$ is large, the null hypothesis will be accepted with a failure to prove independence.

An example of the use of chi square appearAn example of the use of chi square appears in an article by Eden et al. (2008) entitled: *Examining the value of electronic health records on labor and deliver.* [9] In this paperin which the use of an electronic health record (EHR) is was tested in a labor and delivery unit. The chi square test was used to compare documentation quality before and after EHR implementation. Using the distance between O and E before and after, it was found that the chi square value was significantly reduced after the implementation of the EHR [9].

It has been shown that linear regression as a model of statistical analysis is also of great importance to perinatal epidemiology. Logistic regression involves the prediction of outcomes based on a set of numerous variables that may be of numerical or categorical origin. In the case of Peregrine et al., [8] the measured outcome was mode of delivery which was predicted using the following 3 criteria variables: abdominal palpitation of spine position, ultrasonography of head position, and ultrasonography of spine position; all before labor induction. These measurements were all compiled and due to the known increase in cesarean delivery rate for each of these data, it was estimated that the 289 participants of this study would have an 80% probability of a clinically significant increase in observed cesarean delivery rate from 30% (the average rate at this time for the unit where the research was being carried out) to 45%. On an individual basis, one can calculate the probability of an outcome based on a known alteration in the probability of a measured characteristic using the formula: $\frac{1}{1+e^{-z}}$; where z, the increase in probability, is determined from prior studies. When one uses multiple variables in a logistic regression, such as the example above, it is more common to employ the use of a statistical analysis program.

An additional measure of risk, associated with statistical modeling is an odds ratio. This ratio compares of the odds (probability) of an event occurring in two different populations. If the ratio is equal to 1, the event has an equal likelihood of occurring in both populations. An odds ratio greater than one indicates an increase in the probability that the given event will occur in the first population; subsequently, when the ratio is less than one the event is more likely in the second population. The odds ratio can never be less than zero.

In a recent study, odds ratios were employed to demonstrate whether English proficiency and progesterone/estriol levels were found to be correlated with increased odds in preterm birth in acculturated Hispanic populations in the United States of America [10]. An adjusted odds ratio of 4.03 was found for those patients proficient in English, while the lowest quartile of the progesterone/estriol ratio also yielded an increased adjusted odds ratio of 2.93. This means that those patients who spoke English well along with those with lower progesterone/estriol ratios were more likely to have preterm births than those with poorer English skills and higher hormonal ratios.

PRESENTING RESULTS

Once the data have been collected and tested the next step is the presentation of results. There are a variety of ways to present results, however it is important to choose the form which represents the given data in a clear and accurate manner. For example, when one performs an ROC curve it is common to include a line graph which plots the false-positive error rate (x-axis) against sensitivity (y-axis).

Another example of the use of a line graph that involves frequency can be found in figure 1, where the line graph shows birth weight on the x-axis and the percent (frequency) on the y-axis. This is a good way to show descriptive characteristics such as the mode and median birth weights. Figure 6 demonstrates a way to present linear correlation between two variables studied: fetal cheek-to-cheek diameter (CCD), an indicator of subcutaneous tissue mass in the fetus that can be evaluated by ultrasound, and abdominal circumference (AC). The correlation between CCD and the AC is graphically presented below in figure 6 (Pearson correlation coefficient of 0.47; P=0.01). [11].

A simple way of showing frequency of an event is a histogram (figures 2, 3, & 7). For example, one can graph the cases a disease such as idiopathic oligohydramnios and its frequency of occurrence per month (see figure 7). [12] In this case, each month yields a bar whose height is reflective of the quantity of babies born with certain condition. [12] The most common way to display results in medical research is a chart which shows the various percentages, SDs, means or individual values obtained for various variables measured in various populations or sections of a population. This can be seen in nearly all scientific published articles.

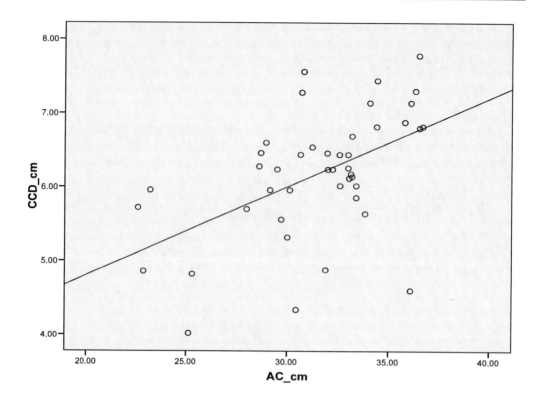

Figure 6. Correlation between the fetal cheek-to-cheek diameter (CCD) and abdominal circumference (AC). [11]

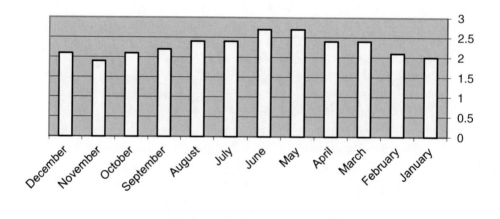

Figure 7. The distribution of cases of idiopathic oligohydramnios during the year. [12]

SAMPLE SIZE DETERMINATION

The sample size, n, is an essential but not sufficient characteristic that constitutes a legitimate scientific study. When designing a study, there are numerous crucial components such as bias-limiting criteria and ethical protocols that contribute to the value and validity of the study. Furthermore, there are standards that must be adhered to in order to verify that the observations made were frequent enough to consider them reflective of a true scientific phenomenon. Fortunately, there are ways to ensure that one has included enough participants in a study to deem one's conclusions generalizable to the greater population.

Firstly, one must determine what it is that he or she would like to prove with a given study. In a prospective study the article *Method of placental removal during cesarean delivery and postpartum complications*, [13], the authors wanted to determine if two methods of placental removal resulted in different rates of postpartum complications such as wound infection and postpartum fever. In order to do so they needed to use two groups of women each exposed to a different type of placental removal. In order to determine how many women would be needed in each group, the following items needed to be considered: what difference (%) should be demonstrated in the outcomes of each groups' treatment, what type of power and what level of statistical significance (probability that results obtained are true) are desired by the researchers.

The first criteria, statistical significance is called "α" or the "p-value." This number comes from what is considered an acceptable type I error rate. Type I errors, ("error of the first kind," an α error, or a "false positive") are false conclusions of differences between two groups being compared, when none exists. This is the error of rejecting a null hypothesis when it is actually true. A type I error in the study above would have been to claim that both methods of placental removal resulted in different postpartum outcomes, when in actuality, no differences existed. As explained above, most commonly a p-value of <0.5 is considered sufficient to prove that any difference seen is most likely reflective of a true phenomenon.

The next component that contributes to sample size is the power that one hopes to achieve in the study. This value comes from what is referred to as 1- β, or one minus the type II error rate. Type II error ("error of the second kind," a β error, or a "false negative") is the error of failing to reject a null hypothesis when it is false. This is the error of failing to observe a difference that exists between two groups. Using the study above as an example, a type II error would have resulted if there was a difference between the amount of postpartum fever and wound infection experienced by those women who received each type of placental removal, when no difference was reported in the study. If the β value (type II error rate) equals the probability of a type II error, then the chance of not performing a type II error is 1-β. An acceptable value for this parameter should also be determined prior to embarking on data collection. The third and final criteria which must be specified in order to determine the sufficient number of participants is the ideal percent difference in outcomes that one would like to find between the two groups being compared. Using these three values, the power of the study, the statistical significance of the study (p-value) and the difference in outcome observable between study groups, one can determine what value of *n* to use in an a study.

In the study mentioned above, it was determined that a minimum of 150 women were needed in each group in order to show a difference in outcome of 15%, a probability of 95%, and a power of 80%. The number referred to as "probability" here, is the chance that a type I error will not occur, the p-value in this case would be 0.05, the standard p-value used in most medical studies.

Once the α value, power and expected difference are known, the actual sample size number usually comes from a chart or most recently comes from an analytical computer program such as PS [14] which calculates power and sample size. One can refer to a sample size chart or a power-analysis program prior to determining the sample size, for instance in the article *Early maternal feeding following caesarean delivery: a prospective randomized* a study, regarding early feeding following cesarean delivery [15] an analytical program was used to determine how many patients would be necessary in each group in order to show a two-fold difference of patient satisfaction (a dichotomous yes/no variable) with a statistical significance of $\alpha = 0.05$ and a power of 80%. This is an example of working backwards from specific goals of power, p-value and ideal difference between groups to determine what sample size would satisfy these criteria. Alternatively, there are situations when only 80 patients are eligible for a specific study and one must use a chart or a power-analysis program in reverse to determine what maximum difference it is possible to demonstrate between groups if each group is comprised of 40 people.

REFERENCES

[1]   Jekel JF, Katz DL, Elmore JG, Wild DMG. *Epidemiology, biostatistics and preventive medicine. 3rd Edition*, Saunders Elsevier, Philadelphia, PA 2007.

[2]   Sheiner E, Mazor-Drey E, Levy A. Asymptomatic bacteriuria during pregnancy. *J Matern Fetal Neonatal Med* 2009 May; 22:423-7.

[3]   Hershkovitz R, Sheiner E, Maymon E, Erez O, Mazor M. Cervical length assessment in women with idiopathic polyhydramnios. *Ultrasound Obstet Gynecol* 2006;4:1-4.

[4]   Sheiner E., Levy A., Katz M., Hershkovitz R., Leron E., Mazor M. Gender Does Matter in Perinatal Medicine. *Fetal Diagnosis and Therapy* 2004; 19:366-369.

[5]   Sheiner E, Shoham-Vardi I, Pombar X, Hussy MJ, Strassner HT, Abramowicz JS. An increased thermal index can be achieved when performing Doppler studies in obstetrical ultrasound. *J Ultrasound Med* 2007;26:71-6.

[6]   Sheiner E, Levy A, Hershokovitz R, Hallak M, Hammel R, Katz M, Mazor M. Determining factors associated with shoulder dystocia: a population-based study. *Eur J Obstet Gynecol Reprod Biol* 2006; 126: 11-5.

[7]   Levy A, Sheiner E, Hammel RD, Hershkovitz H, Hallak M, Katz M, Mazor M. Shoulder dystocia: a comparison of pateints with and without diabetes. *Arch Gynecol Obstet* 2006; 273:203-6.

[8]   Pererine E., O'Brien P., Jauniaux E. Impact on Delivery Outcome of Ultrasonographic Fetal Head Position Prior to Induction of Labor. *Obstet Gynecol* 2007; 109:618-25.

[9]   Eden K, Messina R, Li H, Osterweil P, Henderson C, Guise J. Examining the value of electronic health records on labor and delivery. *Am J Obstet Gynecol.* 2008; 199:307.e1-9.

[10]   Ruiz R. J., Saade G. R., Brown C. E., Nelson-Becker C., Tan A., Bishop S., Bukowski R. The effect of acculturation on progesterone/estriol ratios and preterm birth in Hispanics. *Obstet Gynecol.* 2008;111: 309-16.

[11]   Kerrick H, Sheiner E, Mandell C, Strassner HT, Pombar X, Hussy MJ, Abramowicz JS. The fetal cheek-to-cheek diameter and abdominal circumference: are they correlated? *Arch Gynecol Obstet.* 2009;280:585-8.

[12]   Feldman I, Friger M, Wiznitzer A, Mazor M, Holcberg G, Sheiner E. Is oligohydramnios more common during the summer season? *Arch Gynecol Obstet.* 2009;280:3-6.

[13] Merchavy S, Levy A, Holcberg G, Freedman EN, Sheiner E. Method of placental removal during cesarean delivery and postpartum complications. *Int J Gynaecol Obstet.* 2007;98:232-6.

[14] Dupont WD, Plummer WD: 'Power and Sample Size Calculations: A Review and Computer Program', Controlled Clinical Trials 1990; 11:116-28.

[15] Bar G, Sheiner E, Lezerovizt A, Lazer T, Hallak M. Early maternal feeding following caesarean delivery: a prospective randomised study. *Acta Obstet Gynecol Scand.* 2008;87:68-71.

In: Handbook of Methodological Concepts in Perinatal Medicine ISBN: 978-1-62081-252-5
Editor: Eyal Sheiner © 2013 Nova Science Publishers, Inc.

Chapter 6

INTERPRETATION OF RESEARCH FINDINGS

Ilana Shoham-Vardi[*]

Department of Epidemiology and Health Services Evaluation,
Faculty of Health Sciences, Ben Gurion University of the Negev, Beer Sheva, Israel

INTRODUCTION

Epidemiological studies are designed to assess the association of an exposure and a disease or a clinical condition. Our aim in study design is to obtain the most valid and precise estimate of this association. In interpretation of the data, we are concerned about the extent to which the observed association in our study truly represents the association in the target population, as in most cases we study samples and not entire populations, and even when we do study entire populations we are concerned about whether the findings in this particular population can be generalized to other populations or even to the same population at a different point in time. Our first concern is the likelihood of having made a mistake when deciding to either reject (Type I error) or accept the null hypothesis (Type II error). We use a statistical test to address this concern. This chapter will address further issues of interpretation of research findings. These concerns cannot be left to the stage of data analysis, but should guide the study design at the initial planning stage. All studies have strengths and limitations and researchers should be aware of them when interpreting the study's results. This chapter addresses the issue of validity and the challenges facing the researcher in achieving validity. The readers should be reminded that this chapter is an overview of these rather complex issues as they relate to perinatal research. For a more in-depth discussion, readers are referred to comprehensive epidemiological methods texts such as Rothman [1], Szklow [2] and Kelsey [3].

[*] Tel +972-8-6477453; Fax +972-8-6477638; Email: vilana@bgu.ac.il.

VALIDITY

- *Definition:* The extent to which our tool/instrument/method of measurement actually measures what we intend to measure.

In order to assess validity, we have to decide what is our "gold standard" – i.e the measure which gives us the result that is closest to the truth,—in relation to which we will determine how good is the measurement we have used in our study.

When our measurement is used to assess the presence or absence of a clinical condition or an exposure, and we have a "gold standard", we use the terms *sensitivity* and *specificity* to assess the quality of our measurement:

- *Sensitivity:* The probability that a clinical condition or exposure is correctly assessed as "positive" by our measurement tool.
- *Specificity:* The probability that the absence of a clinical condition or exposure is correctly assessed as "negative" by our measurement tool.
- *Positive predictive value (PPV):* The probability that a case assessed as "positive" actually has the condition
- *Negative predictive value (NPV):* The probability that a case assessed as "negative" actually does not have the condition
-

The concepts of sensitivity, specificity and positive/negative predictive value (PPV) are of particular importance in the context of screening tests, such as prenatal screening for birth defects. The most prevalent prenatal screening test is for Down syndrome. A definitive diagnosis can only be made on the basis of amniocentesis or chorionic villi sampling (CVS). Since these are costly and invasive procedures associated with a certain risk of procedure-related miscarriage, various screening protocols are used to screen and identify women at high risk for Down syndrome and to offer them a diagnostic test. Such screening programs are effective if false positive and false negative rates are low.

In a prospective cohort study of 4373 pregnancies of women who underwent an ultrasound screening for Down syndrome between 16 and 22 weeks of gestation, the validity of two markers of fetal aneuploidy were evaluated: absent or small nasal bone (NB) and increased nuchal fold (NF) (>5 mm and >6 mm). Absent NB was seen in 14/49 cases of Down syndrome for which the NB evaluation was available and NF of >6 mm was seen in 6 of 50 cases (12%) with Down syndrome [4].

Using NF > 5 mm as a cutoff point for a positive screen, six cases out of 50 pregnancies were true positives (TP), while 44 cases of Down syndrome were missed and therefore classified as false negatives (FN). A total of 46 cases had nuchal fold >5 mm, but 40 of those were seen in infants without Down syndrome, thus classified as false positives (FP). Most cases (n= 4283) were truly classified as negative (TN).

Table 1.

Marker	Down Syndrome		
	Yes	No	
Positive (nuchal fold >5 mm)	6 (TP)	40 (FP)	46
Negative (nuchal fold ≤5 mm)	44 (FN)	4283 (TN)	4327
Total	50	4323	4373

We can now calculate the probability that a case of Down syndrome will be detected by our test (Nuchal fold >5 mm), i.e., the sensitivity of the test, expressed as a percentage:

$$SENSITIVITY = \frac{6}{6+44}*100 = 12\%$$

We can calculate the probability that a case without Down syndrome will be correctly classified by our test as normal, i.e., the specificity of the test, expressed as a percentage:

$$SPECIFICITY = \frac{4283}{4283+40}*100 = 99\%$$

We can also ask the question what is the probability that a woman which screened positive (in our example: Nuchal fold >5 mm) actually carries a fetus with Down syndrome?

This probability is a measure called positive predictive value:

$$Positive\ predictive\ value = \frac{TP}{TP+FP}*100$$

$$Positive\ predictive\ value = \frac{6}{6+40}*100 = 13\%$$

The probability that a positive test will actually be diagnosed as Down syndrome is rather low (13%).

Similarly, we can define the predictive value of a negative test:

$$Negative\ predictive\ value = \frac{TN}{TN+FN}*100$$

$$Negative\ predictive\ value = \frac{4283}{4283+44}*100 = 99\%$$

A growing number of epidemiological studies are based on information gathered from large computerized datasets and from national vital statistics computerized records such as birth certificates, notification of infant and fetal deaths, registries of birth defects, registries of very low birth weight infants, etc. The large number of cases, enabling the study of rare conditions and the non-selective population-based nature of such databases are their main advantages. As most of these databases were not originally meant for research purposes, much work has been done to validate the information derived from them [5-8].

RELIABILITY

Often we are unable to truly validate information even when we have information from more than one source, because it is not possible to decide which is a measure that can be considered as the "gold standard". We tend to regard record-based information as superior to self-report, but this is not always justified. Which is a "better" source of information regarding having undergone a certain test in pregnancy: self-report of or data extracted from medical records? Information extracted from medical records will be a more valid source of information if we can be sure that the records contains all tests a patient may have had, as would be the situation if all tests are performed for a given population at a central lab or in a single clinic. Self report may be a more valid source of information in populations where some women may choose to undergo testing in several labs or clinics, not all of which made their records available to us. We need to have good understanding of our sources of information in order to decide which is more valid, but often we do not have enough information to make this decision. In this situation we can ask the question how reliable is the information obtained from these different sources of information, i.e., to what extent is there an agreement between the sources of information. This is also the case when we ask two physicians with the same levels of diagnostic skills to make a diagnosis of the same patient at the same time.

We define reliability as the extent to which information from different sources of information or from repeated measures of the same situation is identical.

The most common clinical situations where reliability is tested are the following:

- *Inter-rater reliability*: In studies based on diagnoses or clinical decisions made by different clinicians or in different study centers, we want to be sure that the same clinical information is interpreted in the same way by the different clinicians at the different sites.
- *Intra*-rater, *or test-retest reliability:* When a new diagnostic skill is introduced or a new research instrument, such as a questionnaire, is considered for use in a study, we want to make sure that the same test or questionnaire results obtained from the same person yield the same results if repeated, under the assumption that no change has occurred between the two measurements.

Statistical tools to assess reliability based on the comparability of two or more sources of information are available. For binary outcomes the most commonly used in the Kappa statistics, and for quantitative measures different types of correlation can be computed. The most commonly used are *Pearson correlation* for normally distributed variables and *Spearman correlation* for ordinal scale variables.

Kappa Statistics

A measure of agreement between two sources of information, adjusted for the proportion of agreement we would expect to occur by chance between those two sources of information.

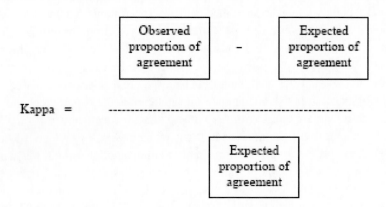

Two sources of information are considered in good agreement if the Kappa statistics are >0.75, fair agreement if Kappa is between 0.75–0.40, and if less than 0.40, poor agreement [9].

Nguyen and Baird [10] compared the reports of both men's and their partner's recall of time to pregnancy, and used the Kappa statistics to assess the reliability of report. The overall Kappa was 0.50 (95% CI 0.40–0.60), i.e., fair agreement.

It is important to note that valid sources of information are reliable; however, even excellent reliability does not necessarily indicate validity. Kelsey [3] gives an example of both man and wife interviewed about drinking habits of the husband. Their reports might be in perfect agreement, but both reports might be totally invalid.

BIAS

The major threat to validity is a study design which leads to systematic wrong estimates of the parameters of interest. Bias in measurement is different from a random error. While random measurement error will on the average yield a correct estimate, bias would give us an estimate that is systemically different from the true value of the parameter.

Bias can result from two sources: a faulty study design where the study population is systematically different from the target population, or from measurement error where the information obtained is systematically different from the truth. The first kind of bias is called selection bias and the second is called information bias. Bias is more likely to occur in retrospective case-control studies than in large, population based studies, but it is possible even in prospective population-based cohort studies.

Selection Bias

Selection bias will occur when the study population is chosen in a way that distorts the true association between the exposure and outcome of interest. In perinatal epidemiology selection bias often occurs when we study populations for whom information is available, which are usually populations who seek medical care, for example women who seek prenatal care. Women can seek prenatal care for a variety of reasons. If one or more of these reasons are unknown to the researchers, and thus unmeasured, is associated with the outcome of interest, we will have a biased estimate of the association between exposure (prenatal care) and pregnancy outcomes. Frick and Lantz [11] present four scenarios leading to a biased estimate of the association between adequate prenatal care and adverse pregnancy outcomes. Favorable Selection: when women with favorable characteristics (for example: high level of education, high income) will be more likely than women with lower level of education or income to seek care and to comply with medical recommendation, and at the same time are more likely to have more favorable birth outcomes, regardless of prenatal care because they lead healthier lifestyles, are less exposed to risk factors such as violence, poor housing conditions, etc., we will overestimate the favorable effect of prenatal care on birth outcome. The opposite will happen if women who are at high risk due to social marginality and possible exposures which will place them at higher risk will not register for prenatal care (Estrangement Selection). Another way selection bias can affect our results is, according to Frick and Lantz [11], Adverse Selection, which will occur if factors that preselect women to prenatal care are risk factors for adverse pregnancy outcomes, such as bad obstetric history, chronic disease, etc. if such selection occurs we are likely to underestimate a favorable effect of prenatal care. If women with no risk factors tend to register late and choose to come for fewer visits (Confidence Selection), will result in underestimate of the effect of prenatal care on birth outcomes.

Selection bias affects cohort studies through selective participation and drop out from follow-up. Even population based data can lead to wrong inferences due to selection bias. Take, for example, epidemiological studies of congenital malformations. Often we use prevalence at birth data and tend to interpret them as if they were incidence data. It has been shown [12] that many pregnancies affected by birth defects tend to result in spontaneous abortions, sometimes in very early pregnancy losses. Moreover, a growing number of birth defects can now be prenatally diagnosed and couples may choose to terminate an affected pregnancy [13-14]. If we compare the prevalence at birth of a certain birth defect in two populations, which differ in the likelihood of prenatal diagnosis and termination of affected pregnancies, we can reach a conclusion that the population which is more likely to carry an affected pregnancy to birth is at higher risk, which is not necessarily true [15]. See, for example, the data in Table 2.

Another example of a selection bias was suggested in a recent study, based on the Texas birth defect registry, on the association between paternal age and birth defects in the offspring. The investigators found that some birth defects in offspring of younger fathers were more likely to be excluded from the database than those of older fathers, thus causing a biased estimate of the association of paternal age and birth defects [8].

Table 2. Percent of Neural Tube Defects (NTD) at birth from all diagnosed cases, by religion, national Israeli data [16]

	JEWS	NON JEWS
Anencephalus	20.3%	39.4%
Spina bifida	20.5%	56.5%

Information Bias

Information bias results from misclassification of disease and/or exposure status caused by faulty measurement tools. This type of bias can affect results of all types of research. Information bias can be either differential or non differential. *Non differential bias* occurs when the information regarding the study outcome variables (disease status in cohort studies, or exposure status in case control studies) is biased in the same direction and magnitude in the compared study groups (exposed and unexposed in cohort studies and in cases and controls in case control studies). Differential bias occurs in cohort studies, if disease status is assessed differently in exposed and unexposed subjects, and in case-control studies if exposure status is assessed differently in cases and controls.

In each situation, the bias will lead to misclassification. Misclassification can occur even when the same assessment method is used, but its validity differs among the study groups. One of the frequent examples of this problem is the use of pregnancy dating methods. It has been shown that using ultrasound for populations with either symmetrically large or small fetuses will be biased [17] For example, fetuses of smokers are known to be symmetrically small, thus the use of ultrasound to date pregnancies of smokers will tend to underestimate gestational age, consequently leading to a possible overestimate of prematurity in smokers [18]. Similarly, bias will occur while comparing rates of preterm birth among populations where different methods of dating are used, or comparing time trends in the rate of pre-term or post-term births when the most common methods of pregnancy dating have been changed [17].

Usually, when information bias affects the two study groups in the same direction and magnitude (non-differential bias), the result will be an underestimate of the true association between disease and exposure—i.e., in a cohort study, the relative risk (RR) and in case-control study, the odds ratio (OR) will be biased toward the null. This type of bias is considered a "conservative bias", if we can still uphold our hypothesis. But sometimes, especially when the association between the exposure and disease is weak and/or the sample size is too small a conservative bias may lead us to a wrong conclusion that there is no association when in fact there is.

When the bias affects each study group differently (differential bias) the effect on the RR or OR will vary according to the direction of the bias in the different study groups.

Recall Bias

Recall bias is a common problem in case-control studies which are based on obtaining information from study participants about past exposures. As at the time of interview the disease status is known, persons with the disease might tend to recall past events and report them more accurately than persons without the disease. Classic examples are case-control studies of birth defects. It has been repeatedly shown, by comparing self reported exposure information to medical records that women who had given birth to an infant with a birth defect tend to report differently than women who had a normal infant. [19]

Interviewer /Observer Bias

Interviewers may be more persistent in their effort to obtain information from cases than from controls. One way to avoid this kind of bias is to keep interviewers as much as possible "blind" to the disease status of the interviewee, or, if that is impossible, interviewers should at least be blind as to the main research hypothesis. [20] Similar problem can occur in cohort studies if different methods are used to assess disease status in exposed and unexposed study participants. For example, if in a prospective cohort study to assess the pregnancy outcomes of women with previous bad obstetric history in comparison with women with normal obstetric history, we follow a cohort of women who enrolled in prenatal care and collect information about pregnancy complications by way of self report in women with bad obstetric history (exposed) and from medical records for women without bad obstetric history (unexposed) an observer bias may occur.

Diagnosis /Detection/Referral Bias

This type of bias is caused when persons with known risks are more likely to be diagnosed, referred and thus diagnosed with the disease than persons without these risk factors, or when persons with a disease are more likely to be tested or questioned about their exposures than persons without the disease. Thus, this type of bias is both a selection and information bias. A recent systematic review examined the evidence of the possible teratogenic effect of paroxetine, a selective serotonin reuptake inhibitor (SSRI) commonly used as an antidepressant by women of childbearing age. The review concluded that the association shown by several studies of first-trimester exposure to paroxetine and an increased risk for cardiac malformations may result from a detection bias, since mothers using SSRIs in pregnancy were more likely to undergo ultrasound in pregnancy and their children were more likely to undergo echocardiograms in the first year of life than children of women who did not use SSRIs. Moreover, more women used the drug for anxiety or panic than women receiving other SSRIs [21].

How to Deal with Bias

Bias, unlike other problems that will be discussed later that may lead to wrong inferences, is caused by faulty study design either in the way the study population is chosen or in the way information is obtained, and therefore it cannot be corrected at the data analysis stage by statistical methods. Thus, careful consideration should be given at the stage of study design to avoid bias as much as possible. Randomized controlled trials (see Chapter 4) are designed to avoid bias, but almost all observational studies are prone to be affected by some sort of bias. It is therefore necessary to collect enough information which can help us to assess the possibility of bias, and to conduct, if necessary, sensitivity analyses, assuming various ways the study findings could have been affected by bias.

CONFOUNDING

The purpose of all epidemiological investigations is to get the best estimate of associations between risk factors (RF) and a disease (D). Confounding is a situation in which a wrong inference about the investigated association between a risk factor (RF) and the disease (D) is made because both RF and D are associated with a third variable that is a true risk factor for the disease. This third variable is called a confounder (C), and its presence can distort the true association between the risk factor and disease under investigation in different ways; it can cause a nonexisting association between RF and D to appear as if there is an association, and it can cause an existing association to disappear, but most frequently confounding causes over- or underestimation of a true association.

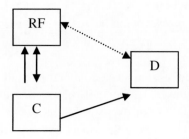

Unlike bias, which results from a faulty study design, confounding is caused by our inability, in observational studies, to take apart into simple components a complex reality. How can we test the effect of very young maternal age per se on birth outcomes in the US, where most teenage pregnancies are often characterized by unhealthy behaviors and limited access to health services characteristics that in and of themselves were shown to be associated with adverse pregnancy outcomes? Or, how can we test the effect of strenuous work in pregnancy on length of gestation if most pregnant women who hold physically strenuous jobs during pregnancy are exposed to other risk factors such as poverty, single motherhood and low level of education? One way is to study the relationship in populations where the exposure of interest is not associated with other known risk factors. An example is the study of Klebanoff, Shiono and Rhodas [22] on the association between strenuous work in pregnancy and preterm birth where the population exposed to physically strenuous work were pregnant female medical residents and the "unexposed" were pregnant wives of male residents. The researchers' conclusion that "working long hours in a stressful occupation has little effect on the outcome of pregnancy in an otherwise healthy population of high socioeconomic status" suggested that association between physical work and preterm birth reported in earlier studies might have been confounded by socioeconomic and other risk factors.

Another approach is to control for the confounding factors in appropriate statistical methods either by stratification (bivariate analysis) or by multivariable regression analyses. Stratified analysis allows the researcher to examine the pattern of association between the exposure of interest and the outcome in varying levels of the suspected confounder variable. If the same pattern of association is observed, it is possible to use the Mantel Haenszel technique to calculate an adjusted measure of association (relative risk or odds ratio). In a study comparing the risk of caesarian section (CS) in older primiparae (age>40) who conceived spontaneously and those who conceived by reproductive assisted technique, the authors conducted a stratified analysis to control for a variety of risk factors that may have been associated with both infertility and with indications for CS and found that, regardless of clinical conditions, nulliparous women who conceived after infertility treatment had an increased risk for CS delivery [23].

If different patterns of association are observed at different levels of the confounding variable, we conclude that an interaction, or effect modification, exists between the confounder variable and the exposure under study. A recent example was reported in a retrospective cohort study of twins of whom only one survived and the other died either intrapartum or neonatally [24]. The purpose of the study was to determine whether birth order is associated with mortality risk. While no association between birth order and the overall risk was found, birth order was found to significantly interact with gestational age. Among preterm deliveries, there was no association between birth order and risk of mortality, but in term deliveries the second twin was at a markedly increased risk of dying from intrapartum anoxia or trauma.

Multivariable regression analyses are used to control simultaneously for several potential confounders. Thus, the measures of association obtained from a multivariable regression represents the unique association of our exposure of interest and the outcome variable when all other confounder variables included in the model are held constant. Various multivariable regression models were developed to be applied for different research questions. (See chapter 7 for a detailed discussion of multivariable analysis.)

REFERENCES

[1]   Rothman K.J., Greenland S., & Lash T.L. (2008). *Modern Epidemiology,* 3rd Edition. Philadelphia, PA: Lippincott, Williams & Wilkins.
[2]   Szklow M. & Nieto FJ. (2007) *Epidemiology Beyond the Basics*, 2nd Edition. Sudbury MA, Jones and Bartlett Publishers.
[3]   Kelsey J. *Methods in Observational Epidemiology*, 2nd Edition 1996 Oxford University Press, Incorporated.
[4]   Odibo AO, Sehdev HM, Gerkowicz S, Stamilio DM, Macones GA: Comparison of the efficiency of second-trimester nasal bone hypoplasia and increased nuchal fold in Down syndrome screening. *Am J Obstet Gynecol.* 2008;199(3):281.e1-5
[5]   Melve KK, Lie RT, Skjaerven R, Van Der Hagen CB, Gradek GA, Jonsrud C, Braathen GJ, Irgens LM. Registration of Down syndrome in the Medical Birth Registry of Norway: validity and time trends. *Acta Obstet Gynecol Scand.* 2008;87(8):824-30.

[6]   Ford JB, Roberts CL, Algert CS, Bowen JR, Bajuk B, Henderson-Smart DJ; NICUS group.Using hospital discharge data for determining neonatal morbidity and mortality: avalidation study. *BMC Health Serv Res.* 2007 Nov 20;7:188

[7]   Lydon-Rochelle MT, Cárdenas V, Nelson JL, Tomashek KM, Mueller BA, Easterling TR. Validity of maternal and perinatal risk factors reported on fetal death certificates. *Am J Public Health.* 2005 Nov;95 (11):1948-51. Epub 2005.

[8]   Archer NP, Langlois PH, Suarez L, Brender J, Shanmugam R. Association of paternal age with prevalence of selected birth defects. *Birth Defects Res A Clin Mol Teratol.* 2007 Jan;79(1):27-34.

[9]   Fleiss JL. *Statistical methods for rates and proportions,* 2nd ed. New York, NY, John Wiley and Sons, 1981

[10]   Nguyen RH, Baird DD.Accuracy of men's recall of their partner's time to pregnancy. *Epidemiology.* 2005 Sep;16(5):694-8.

[11]   Frick KD. Lantz PM. Selection Bias in prenatal care utilization: An interdisciplinary framework and review of the literature. *Med Care Res Rev* 1996:53: 371-96.

[12]   Rivas F, Dávalos IP, Olivares N, Dávalos NO, Pérez-Medina R, Gómez-Partida G,Chakraborty R.Reproductive history in mothers of children with neural tube defects. *Gynecol Obstet Invest.* 2000;49(4):255-60.

[13]   Cragan JD, Roberts HE, Edmonds LD, Khoury MJ, Kirby RS, Shaw GM, Velie EM, Merz RD, Forrester MB, Williamson RA, Krishnamurti DS, Stevenson RE, Dean JH. Surveillance for anencephaly and spina bifida and the impact of prenatal diagnosis— United States, 1985-1994. *MMWR CDC Surveill Summ.* 1995;44(4):1-13.

[14]   Van Allen MI, Boyle E, Thiessen P, McFadden D, Cochrane D, Chambers GK, Langlois S, Stathers P, Irwin B, Cairns E, MacLeod P, Delisle MF, Uh SH. The impact of prenatal diagnosis on neural tube defect (NTD) pregnancy versus birth incidence in British Columbia. *Appl Genet.* 2006;47(2):151-8.

[15]   Zlotogora J, Amitai Y, Kaluski DN, Leventhal A. Surveillance of neural tube defects in Israel. *Isr Med Assoc J.* 2002;4(12):1111-4.

[16]   Department for community genetics. Public Health Services, Ministry of Health. Israel. *Open Neural Birth Defects in Israel.* Jerusalem September 2002.

[17]   Lynch CD, Zhang J The research implications of the selection of a gestational age estimation method. *Paediatr Perinat Epidemiol.* 2007 Sep;21 Suppl 2:86-96.

[18]   Horta BL, Victora CG, Menezes AM, Halpern R, Barros FC: Low birthweight, preterm births and intrauterine growth retardation in relation to maternal smoking. *Paediatr Perinat Epidemiol.* 1997;11(2):140-51.

[19]   Rockenbauer M, Olsen J, Czeizel AE, Pedersen L, Sørensen HT; EuroMAP Group. Recall bias in a case-control surveillance system on the use of medicine during pregnancy. *Epidemiology.* 2001 Jul;12 (4):461-6.

[20]   Watson LF, Lumley J, Rayner JA, Potter A.Research interviewers' experience in the Early Births study of very preterm birth: qualitative assessment of data collection processes in a case-control study. *Paediatr Perinat Epidemiol.* 2007 Jan;21(1):87-94.

[21]   Bar-Oz B, Einarson T, Einarson A, Boskovic R, O'Brien L, Malm H, Bérard A, Koren G.Paroxetine and congenital malformations: meta-Analysis and consideration of potential confounding factors. *Clin Ther.* 2007 May;29(5):918-26.

[22]   Klebanoff MA, Shiono PH, Rhoads GG. Outcomes of pregnancy in a national sample of resident physicians. *N Engl J Med.* 1990 Oct 11;323(15):1040-5.

[23] Sheiner E, Shoham-Vardi I, Hershkovitz R, Katz M, Mazor M. Infertility treatment is an independent risk factor for cesarean section among nulliparous women aged 40 and above. *Am J Obstet Gynecol.* 2001;185:888-92.

[24] Smith GC, Fleming KM, White IR. Birth order of twins and risk of perinatal death related to delivery in England, Northern Ireland, and Wales, 1994-2003: retrospective cohort study. *BMJ.* 2007;334 (7593):576.

In: Handbook of Methodological Concepts in Perinatal Medicine   ISBN: 978-1-62081-252-5
Editor: Eyal Sheiner   © 2013 Nova Science Publishers, Inc.

Chapter 7

THE IMPORTANCE OF MULTIVARIABLE ANALYSIS FOR CONDUCTING AND EVALUATING RESEARCH IN PERINATOLOGY

Mitchell H. Katz[*]

Los Angeles Department of Health Services
Los Angeles, CA, US

INTRODUCTION

Multivariable analysis is essential to the study of perinatology. Why? Because many of the important outcomes in the field of perinatology for example, pre-eclampsia, prematurity, infants born small for gestational age, periventricular hemorrhage have multiple interrelated causes. Therefore, studies aimed at understanding and ultimately preventing negative outcomes and promoting successful ones must use multivariable analysis. Moreover, it is not just researchers who must be familiar with these models. As the number of articles using multivariable analysis increases in the literature, clinicians and other readers must be sufficiently familiar with the models to correctly interpret and apply the results.

Unfortunately, it is impossible to do justice to the topic of multivariable analysis in a single chapter. That's why I have written a book about it. [1] It is possible, however, to answer a number of key questions about multivariable analyses. In doing so, I have focused on examples from the perinatology literature in the hope that it will make the explanations more relevant for perinatologists.

WHAT IS MULTIVARIABLE ANALYSIS?

Multivariable analysis is a statistical tool for determining the unique contributions of a variety of factors to a single event or outcome. For example, a variety of factors are

[*] Email: mkatz@dhs.lacounty.gov.

associated with delivery of an infant small for gestational age, including maternal age, nulliparity, smoking, ethnicity, and administration of steroids. Depending on the context, these factors are referred to as risk factors, independent variables, explanatory variables, or treatment/intervention effects. Multivariable analysis enables us to determine the *independent* contribution of each of these risk factors to an outcome, such as the occurrence of an infant small for gestational age. (Outcome may also be referred to as the dependent variable or the response variable).

WHY IS MULTIVARIABLE ANALYSIS NEEDED?

There are four major reasons for performing multivariable analysis (Table 1).

Table 1. Why is multivariable analysis needed?

	Examples
Identify the unique contribution of a variety of risk factors to a single outcome.	Genital HSV infection, lack of antiretroviral prophylaxis, increased duration of membrane rupture, and increased gestational age are all independent risk factors for perinatal transmission of HIV. [2]
Identify and adjust for confounding	Pre-term delivery appeared to be associated with a higher rate of intraventricular hemorrhage because the association was confounded by gestational age. [3]
Develop a diagnostic/prognostic model	A logistic regression model using estimated fetal weight and the ductus venosus pulsatility correctly predicted a poor outcome in 66.7% of the cases of infants born to mothers with pre-eclampsia and a good outcome in 98.0% of the cases with an overall accuracy of 94.5%. [5]
Adjust models for variation in risk groups within treatment groups	Even in the absence of confounding, when using a non-linear model, adjust for baseline characteristics to avoid incorrect estimates of treatment effect.

First, to better understand and improve outcomes in perinatology, it is important to identify unique risk factors for positive and negative outcomes. For example, Chen and colleagues assessed risk factors for perinatal transmission of the human immunodeficiency virus. [2]

As you can see in Table 2, a bivariate analysis shows that there are four significant predictors of perinatal transmission: genital herpes simplex (HSV) infection during pregnancy, lack of zidovudine prophylaxis, a long delay in membrane rupture, and greater gestational age at delivery. But are these risk factors independent of one another? Does each contribute to an increase risk of HIV transmission or is it possible that some of the risk factors are redundant with one another (e.g., patients with HSV infection are also less likely to take zidovudine prophylaxis)?

Answering this question requires multivariable analysis. Indeed, a multiple logistic regression (Table 3) indicates that each of these four variables contributes to HIV transmission. The analysis leads us to believe that to prevent perinatal transmission we should avoid or minimize all four of these risk factors.

Table 2. Bivariate Risk Factors for Perinatal transmission of HIV

Maternal Variable	No. of Women*	No. of Infected Infants (%)	Odds Ratio	95% Confidence Interval	P
Diagnosis of genital HSV infection during pregnancy					
Yes	21	6 (28.6)	3.4	1.3-9.3	.02
No	381	40 (10.5)			
Lack of zidovudine prophylaxis during pregnancy / delivery					
Yes	124	21 (16.9)	2.0	1.1-3.7	.04
No	266	25 (9.4)			
Duration of membrane rupture (h)					
≥4	151	29 (19.2)	3.0	1.6-5.7	.001
<4	217	16 (7.4)			
Gestational age at delivery (wk)					
< 37	66	18 (27.3)	4.0	2.0-7.8	<.001
≥ 37	327	28 (8.6)			

* Numbers for some variables do not add up to total because of missing data.
Data from Chen KT, Segúu M, Lumey LH, et al. Genital herpes simplex virus infection and perinatal transmission of human immunodeficiency virus. *Obstet Gynecol*. 2005;106:1341-8.

Table 3. Risk Factors for Perinatal Transmission of HIV

Risk Factor	Adjusted OR	95% CI	P
Diagnosis of genital HSV infection during pregnancy	4.8	1.3-17.0	.02
Lack of zidovudine prophylaxis during pregnancy/ delivery	2.2	1.1-4.4	.02
Rupture of membranes ≥4 hours	2.5	1.3-5.0	.01
Delivery at < 37 weeks of gestation	3.4	1.6-7.0	.001

Data from Chen KT, Segúu M, Lumey LH, et al. Genital herpes simplex virus infection and perinatal transmission of human immunodeficiency virus. *Obstet Gynecol*. 2005;106:1341-8.

In addition to identifying the unique contribution of different risk factors to a particular outcome, a second important function of multivariable analysis is to identify and adjust for *confounding*. Confounding occurs when the apparent association between a risk factor and an outcome is affected by the relationship of a third variable to the risk factor and to the outcome; the third variable is called a confounder. To be a confounder, a variable must be *associated with* the risk factor and *causally related to* the outcome (Figure 1).

To illustrate how multivariable analysis enables us to identify and adjust for confounding, let's examine the data from a study assessing whether outcomes are different for infants who have an indicated preterm delivery compared to those who had a spontaneous preterm delivery among neonates weighing < 1000 grams at birth. [3] The most common reasons for indicated preterm delivery were severe preeclampsia or eclampsia.

It would appear from the bivariate data shown in Table 4 that infants with indicated preterm delivery were less likely to have intraventricular hemorrhage than those with spontaneous preterm delivery. The 95% confidence interval for the bivariate odds ratio of 0.35 excludes 1, indicating that the association is statistically significant. However, infants who had an indicated preterm delivery were at a greater mean gestational age (28 weeks) than those with spontaneous preterm delivery (26 weeks).

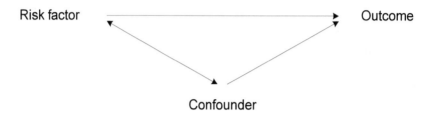

Figure 1. Relationship among risk factor, confounder, and outcome. [Reprinted with permission from Katz, MH. Multivariable Analysis: A Practical Guide for Clinicians (2nd edition). Cambridge: Cambridge University Press, 2006.]

Table 4. Does indicated pre-term delivery decrease neonatal morbidity in infants <1000 grams?

	Intraventricular hemorrhage (III/IV)		
	Yes	No	Total
Indicated pre-term delivery	9 (5.8 %)	147 (94.2 %)	156
Spontaneous pre-term delivery	38 (14.9%)	217 (85.1 %)	255
	47	364	411
OR = 0.35 (0.16 – 0.76)			

Data from Kimberlin DF, et al. Indicated versus spontaneous preterm delivery: An evaluation of neonatal morbidity among infants weighing ≤1000 grams at birth. *Am J Obstet Gynecol* 1999;180:683-9.

When the investigators performed a multivariable logistic regression adjusting for gestational age they found that the difference in the frequency of intraventricular hemorrhage between those infants born following indicated preterm delivery and those born following spontaneous preterm delivery became smaller (odds ratio of 0.66) and the confidence intervals did not exclude one (0.34 – 1.31). In other words, the outcomes did not differ based on whether preterm delivery is indicated or spontaneous. What happened? Gestational age is confounding the association between indicated preterm delivery and intraventricular hemorrhage (Figure 2).

Multivariable analysis is not the only statistical method for identifying and eliminating confounding. Stratified analysis also can be used to assess the effect of a risk factor on an outcome while holding other variables constant, thereby eliminating confounding. However, stratification works well only in situations where there are only one or two confounders. When there are many potential confounders, as is usually the case is perinatology, stratifying the sample for all possible confounders will create literally hundreds of groups in which the investigators would need to determine the relationship between the risk factor and the outcome. Because the sample sizes would be small, the estimates of risk would be unstable.

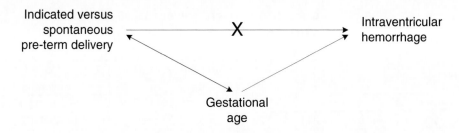

Figure 2. Gestational age confounds the relationship between indicated pre-term delivery and intraventricular hemorrhage.

Given this discussion of the importance of multivariable analysis for minimizing confounding you may assume that you would not have to use multivariable analysis for a randomized controlled trial. After all, randomization produces unbiased groups; since group assignment is determined randomly it cannot be influenced by factors that favor one group over the other(s). Therefore differences between the groups, in response to an intervention, cannot be due to how the groups were assembled.

However, the reality is that the majority of randomized controlled trials perform multivariable analysis for one of a variety of reasons. First, it is possible that by chance (bad luck!) the randomized study groups differ on an important baseline characteristic. In this circumstance, you would use multivariable analysis to adjust for the difference. Second, even if the groups appear to be balanced, there may be small differences that together could bias your study. In some ways, adjusting for baseline differences using a multivariable model has become the standard of demonstrating that there is no confounding. If the unadjusted and the adjusted rates are the same, then you have evidence that there is no confounding due to these measured characteristics. Third, investigators may perform multivariable analysis in the context of a randomized controlled trial to identify additional independent predictors of outcome other than the randomized treatment. This is akin to using multivariable analysis to identify the unique contribution of a variety of risk factors to a single cause.

To illustrate the uses of multivariable analysis within a randomized study, let's look at a randomized controlled trial comparing the effect of preoperative vaginal preparation with povidone-iodine versus the standard abdomen only scrub on the rate of post-cesarean endometritis. [4] In a bivariate analysis women who received the vaginal scrub were significantly less likely to develop endometritis following cesarean section (odds ratio = 0.45; 95% confidence intervals 0.21-0.97). Since this was a randomized trial there should be no confounding. The authors checked to see if there were baseline differences between those subjects in the treatment group and those in the placebo group. None were statistically significant. However, there were some non-significant differences between the groups that could bias the estimate of the effect of a vaginal preparation on the rate of endometritis. Therefore the authors performed a multivariable analysis (shown in Table 5). As you can see, with adjustment for severe anemia, use of intrapartum internal monitors, and history of antenatal genitourinary infections, vaginal rub was protective for endometritis. The odds ratio (0.44) from the multivariate model was practically identical to that of the bivariate analysis, indicating that there was not confounding due to the other variables that were in the model. The fact that the other three variables in Table 5 were statistically significant indicates that these variables are also unique contributors to endometritis.

**Table 5. Multivariate Analysis of Factors Affecting Risk
for Postcesarean Endometritis (N=308)**

Variable	Adjusted Odds Ratio	95% Confidence Interval
Vaginal scrub	0.44	0.193-0.997
Severe anemia (hematocrit <30%)	4.26	1.568-11.582
Use of intrapartum internal monitors	2.84	1.311-6.136
History of antenatal genitourinary infections	2.89	1.265-6.595

Data from Starr R, et al. Preoperative vaginal preparation with povidone-Iodine and the risk of postcesarean endometritis. *Obstet Gynecol.* 2005;105:1024-9.

A third reason to perform multivariable analysis is to develop a model containing multiple variables that can be used to diagnose conditions or to provide prognostic information about a particular condition. For example, Geerts and Odentaal used multiple logistic regression to predict a poor outcome in infants of women with pre-eclampsia. [5] A poor outcome was defined as perinatal mortality or evidence of neurologic compromise of the infant at discharge. The investigators found that the best model for predicting poor outcome was the combination of initial estimated fetal weight and final ductus venosus pulsatility index. It had a correct prediction of poor outcome in 66.7% of the cases, good outcome in 98.0% of the cases, and overall accuracy of 94.5%.

There are several differences between predictive/prognostic models and the explanatory models that we have been discussing so far. With predictive/prognostic models we are not as interested in the individual variables; in fact, it doesn't matter whether the variables are causally related to the outcome or not. Instead we are interested in how well the model predicts the outcome in a variety of settings; as is the case with the study by Geerts and Odentall, [5] some of the variables (e.g., pulsatility index) may be diagnostic tests rather than risk factors that are causally related to the outcome.

Table 6. Type of outcome variable determines choice of multivariable analysis

Type of outcome	Example of outcome variable	Type of multivariable analysis
Interval	Gestational Weight	Multiple linear regression Analysis of variance
Dichotomous	Pre-eclampsia (Y/N)	Multiple logistic regression
Ordinal	Grade of intraventricular hemorrhage	Proportional odds regression
Nominal	Pre-term Pre-eclampsia, term Pre-eclampsia, small for gestational age neonate, normal pregnancy	Polytomous logistic regression
Time to occurrence of a dichotomous event	Establish prenatal care	Proportional hazards analysis
Rare outcomes and counts	Birth defects	Poisson regression

A fourth reason for conducting multivariable analysis is that variation in subjects' risk factors within study groups can result in incorrect estimates of the treatment effect in nonlinear models (e.g., logistic or proportional hazard regression) even when risk factors are balanced between the study groups. [6] In such cases, adjusting for risk factors in a multivariable model will yield more accurate estimates of the treatment effect.

WHAT TYPES OF MULTIVARIABLE ANALYSIS ARE COMMONLY USED IN PERINATAL RESEARCH?

Commonly used methods of multivariable analysis are shown in Table 6. As you can see the type of multivariable analysis to perform depends on the type of outcome variable you are using.

Linear regression and analysis of variance are used with interval (also called continuous) outcomes (e.g., gestational age). With interval variables, equal sized differences on all parts of the scale are equal. Gestational age is an interval variable because the difference between an age of 30 and 33 (3 weeks) is the same as the difference between an age of 33 and 36 (3 weeks).

Logistic regression is used with dichotomous outcomes (e.g., pre-eclampsia (yes/no)). Dichotomous variables, as implied by the name, are those variables that have only two values, such as yes/no, dead/alive.

Ordinal variables are analyzed using proportional odds regression. An ordinal variable has multiple values that can be "ordered" but unlike an interval variable there is not an equal size difference on each part of the scale. The difference between grade I and III intraventricular hemorrhage and II and IV ventricular hemorrhage is not the same amount of hemorrhage.

Nominal variables are analyzed using polytomous logistic regression. Nominal variables are categorical variables that cannot be ordered. They represent different states. For examples, Erez and colleagues used polytomous logistic regression to compare possible outcomes: delivery of a small for neonate gestational age, pre-term eclampsia, term eclampsia, and normal pregnancy. [7]

Proportional hazards regression is used when we are interested in the length of time to reach a discrete event (e.g., survival time). For example, Wy and colleagues used proportional hazards regression to identify neonatal and maternal predictors of death in infants born with a diagnosis of Hydrops Fetalis. [8] Poisson regression is used for rare outcomes such as birth defects or for analyzing the rates of outcomes (e.g., rates of pregnancies in a community over time).

WHAT INDEPENDENT VARIABLES SHOULD I ENTER INTO A MULTIVARIABLE ANALYSIS?

For explanatory models each multivariable model should include the risk factor(s) and potential confounders. However, deciding which potential confounders to include is neither standard nor straightforward.

Ideally researchers should include in their models all those variables that have been hypothesized on theoretical grounds or shown in prior research to be confounders of the relationship being studied.

Although researchers should err on the side of including potentially important variables in the analysis, it is important to exclude extraneous ones. For example, seat belt usage should not be included in a model predicting early initiation of prenatal care, even though it may well be associated with this outcome. The reason is that seat belt use is not a potential cause of initiating prenatal care. It just happens that people who are more likely to comply with seat belts are also more likely to comply with recommendations about when to initiate prenatal care.

It is also important to exclude variables that are on the causal pathway of an outcome; these variables are referred to as intervening variables. For example, if you are testing the effectiveness of antiretroviral treatment on reducing the likelihood of transmission of the human immunodeficiency virus (HIV) from an infected mother to her fetus, it would be a mistake to include the change in the maternal viral load between initiation of treatment and delivery. Why? Because one of the mechanisms by which antiretroviral treatment prevents perinatal transmission is by reducing maternal viral load (Figure 3). If you adjust for the decrease in viral load, you will be adjusting away the effect you are trying to demonstrate. Of course, it would be okay to include maternal viral load prior to treatment as a risk factor in a model predicting treatment efficacy. It would also be okay to perform two models evaluating treatment efficacy with and without adjustment for change in maternal viral load. Comparison of the models would show how much of the effect of antiretroviral treatment is due to the effect of treatment on maternal viral load and how much is due to other ways that antiretroviral treatment prevents infection. For example, Sperling and colleagues, using a logistic regression model, estimated that decrease in viral load explained 17% of the treatment effect of zidovudine in preventing perinatal transmission. [9]

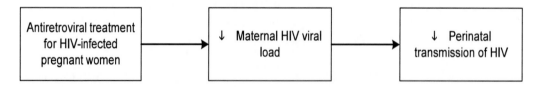

Figure 3. Maternal viral HIV viral load is an intervening variable between antiretroviral treatment and perinatal transmission.

When there are variables in the data set that are highly correlated to each other, you should include only one. The reason is that when two variables are highly correlated it is impossible for the model to identify the independent contribution of each a problem referred to as *multicollinearity*. For example, in a study of neonatal mortality, the investigators found that birth weight and gestational age were too closely related to one another to include both in the model. [10] They excluded gestational age because it had more missing data than birth weight.

After excluding extraneous variables, intervening variables, and redundant variables, you still may have too many variables in your model for your sample size. This can result in unreliable estimates and wide confidence intervals. As a rule of thumb, to have confidence in the results, there should be at least 20 subjects per independent variable eligible for inclusion into a linear regression model, and at least ten outcomes per independent variable eligible for inclusion into a logistic regression or proportional hazards model. [11-13] Sample size requirements for logistic regression and proportional hazards regression are expressed as outcomes per variable (rather than subjects per variable). The needed sample size is based on the less frequent state of the outcome. If only six babies suffer fetal demise, the model will have difficulty predicting how three variables independently predict demise even if there are 994 normal births.

Wide confidence intervals are a consequence of an insufficient sample size. Whenever you see confidence intervals that are clinically meaningless (risk between 0.8 and 22.0), it is likely that the sample size is insufficient for answering the question.

There are several techniques you can use to decrease the number of variables in your model. As discussed above, you should remove variables that are extraneous to your theory. Sometimes you can combine more than one variable into a scale. For example, education, income, ethnicity, and geographic location may be satisfactorily summarized by a variable measuring socioeconomic status. Another technique is to empirically test individual variables to determine whether they are confounders. Even if a variable is theoretically thought to be a confounder, if inclusion of the variable in the model makes no difference to the estimate of the risk between the independent variable(s) and the outcome of interest, it is not empirically functioning as a confounder and can potentially be excluded. [1]

It is also possible to reduce the number of variables in a model using automatic variable selection algorithms. These algorithms allow the computer to choose what variables to include in the model based on specific criteria. Variable selection methods include: *forward stepwise selection* (the variable with the strongest association with the outcome enters first, followed by the next strongest until all variables that are related to outcome, at an investigator specified significance level, have entered the model; if any of the variables that entered the model are no longer significant when the other variables are in the model, they will be sequentially deleted); *backward deletion* (all variables enter the model and are sequentially deleted starting with the variable having the weakest association with the outcome and continuing until the only variables left in the model are those related to outcome at an investigator specified level); and *best subset* (the subset of variables that maximizes the specifications chosen by the researcher).

Although, automatic variable selection techniques often produce models with a smaller number of independent variables, they have many serious limitations and should be avoided. [14-16] The variables that are retained in a model using automatic algorithms are not necessarily clinically more important than the variables that are excluded. If two variables are significantly associated with one another, the model will likely choose the one with the better statistical characteristics. It is much better for the investigator rather than the computer to determine which variables should be kept and which variables should be deleted.

IN WHAT FORM SHOULD INDEPENDENT VARIABLES BE ENTERED INTO A MULTIVARIABLE MODEL?

To enter an independent variable into a multivariable model it should be in the form of an interval or dichotomous variable. Nominal variables can never be entered in their original form. Instead, to enter a nominal variable into a multivariable model you must create multiple dichotomous variables (also referred to as "*dummy*" variables) to represent it. For example, the variable ethnicity, might be represented with four variables: Caucasian (yes/no), African-American (yes/no), Latino (yes/no), Asian (yes/no), with mixed ethnicity or other ethnicity as the reference group.

WHAT ASSUMPTIONS UNDERLIE MULTIVARIABLE MODELS?

Multivariable models are mathematical expressions. We choose particular models because we believe that the data will follow the form of that model. If the model does not fit the data, our understanding of the data will be distorted.

The underlying assumption of multiple linear regression is that as the independent variables increase (or decrease), the mean value of the outcome increases (or decreases) in a linear fashion. Although the relationship between the independent variable and the outcome must be linear, it is possible to model non-linear relationships by transforming the variables so that the independent variables have a linear relationship to the outcome. Readers will commonly see the use of logarithmic and spline transformations to model nonlinear relationships.

Logistic regression models the probability of an outcome, and how that probability changes with a change in the predictor variables. The basic assumption is that each one unit increase in a predictor multiplies the odds of the outcome by a certain factor (the odds ratio of the predictor), and that the effect of several variables is the multiplicative product of their individual effects. The logistic function produces a probability of outcome bounded by 0 and 1.

Proportional hazards models assume that the ratio of the hazard functions for persons with and without a given risk factor is the same over the entire study period. This is known as the *proportionality assumption*. [1, 17-19]

A major advantage of proportional hazards analysis is that it allows incorporation of subjects with varying lengths of follow-up. Varying lengths of follow-up occur commonly in longitudinal studies for several reasons including subjects being lost to follow-up, subjects developing a condition that makes it impossible to evaluate them for the study's outcome of interest, and subjects being enrolled in waves, resulting in some subjects having longer lengths of follow-up than other subjects. [20] Subjects who have not experienced the outcome of interest by the end of the study are referred to as censored observations.

In proportional hazards analyses censored subjects are assumed to have had the same course, if they hadn't been censored, as subjects who were not censored. In other words, the losses occur randomly, independent of outcome. It is this assumption that allows us to incorporate the follow-up time of censored subjects in the analysis. However, sometimes losses occur due to a systematic bias such as when persons who are lost to follow-up are more likely to have experienced the outcome of interest than those persons not lost to follow-up.

All of the multivariable statistics discussed thus far assume that observations are independent of one another; that is, the outcome for one subject is not influenced by the outcome of another subject. But in some perinatology studies the outcomes of some subjects may be correlated to each other (also referred to as clustered observations). For example, in a study of birth outcomes, some pregnancies will result in multiple births. It would not be correct to treat twins as two independent observations because they share the same mother and therefore the same physiology and depending on whether they are identical or fraternal twins, 50-100% of the genetics.

Although twinning may be the most obvious example of non-independent observations in the field of perinatology, there are a number of situations where observations may not be independent. For example, repeated observations of the same person (e.g., outcomes of different pregnancies) are not independent; we would expect that the second pregnancy of a woman would more closely resemble her first pregnancy than the pregnancy of a different woman. Also, women drawn from the same obstetrics practice are more likely to be similar to each other than women drawn from different practices.

When you have clustered observations, you need a multivariable technique that can incorporate clustered observations. Two such techniques are: *generalized estimating equations* and *mixed-effects models* (also known as mixed models, random effects regression models, random coefficient models, multilevel models and hierarchical models). [1, 21, 22]

How Should Interactions between Independent Variables be Interpreted?

An *interaction* occurs when the effect of a risk factor on an outcome is changed by the value of a third variable. As illustrated in Figure 4 the risk factor's effect on outcome (solid lines) differs depending on the value of the interaction variable. Note how the dotted line is the average of the two effects. Because the value of the third variable changes the effect of the risk on an outcome, interaction is often referred to as effect modification.

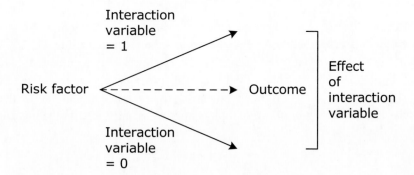

Figure 4. Illustration of an interaction effect. [Reprinted with permission from Katz, MH. Multivariable Analysis: A Practical Guide for Clinicians (2nd edition). Cambridge: Cambridge University Press, 2006.]

Interactions are different from confounding in that with interactions the relationship between the risk factor and the outcome is not due a third variable; rather the relationship varies depending on the value of the third variable. For example, Smith and colleagues assessed the ability of pregnancy-associated plasma protein A and alpha-fetoprotein in predicting preterm birth. [23] In a multivariate logistic model with the outcome of preterm delivery they entered two variables: pregnancy related plasma protein A and alpha-fetoprotein; the odds ratio associated with a low plasma protein A was 2.2 and the odds ratio associated with a high alfa-fetoprotein was 2.1. Because odds ratios in a logistic regression model have a multiplicative effect on outcome, the model containing these two variables would predict that a mother with an low plasma protein A level and a high alfa-fetoprotein level would have a risk of preterm delivery of 4.6 (2.2 x 2.1).

However, the reality was more complicated. The increase in risk was much higher in patients with both a low plasma protein A level and a high alfa-fetoprotein level than predicted by the product (4.6) of the odds ratios. The actual odds ratio for this group was 9.9. There was an interaction. The combination of a low plasma protein A level and a high alfa-fetoprotein level resulted in a higher risk of preterm delivery than you would think from the odds ratios of the individual variables. Interactions can be diagnosed by looking at the risk associated with different subgroups (e.g., the odds ratio associated with having only a low plasma protein A level, the odds ratio associated with having only a high alfa-fetoprotein level, and the odds ratio associated with having both risk factors). Interactions can also be diagnosed by entering into a multiple regression analysis the individual variables along with a product term. In the case of this example, you would enter plasma protein level (coded as 1 for low and 0 for high), alfa-fetoprotein level (coded as 0 for low and 1 for high) and the product term (plasma protein level x alfa-feto protein level).

Although the search for interactions can be clinically meaningful, as was the case in this study, readers should be skeptical of interaction terms that are not specified *a priori*. The reason is that when investigators search for interactions they are essentially performing subgroup analyses. The more interactions searched for, the more subgroups tested, and the greater the possibility that the relationship between the dependent variable and the outcome will differ, due to chance, in one or more of the different subgroups.

DOES THE MODEL FIT THE DATA?

The best way to assess whether the model fits the data is through residual analysis. *Residuals* are the difference between the observed and the estimated value. [1, 24] They can be thought of as the error in estimation. Large residuals suggest that the model does not fit the data. It may be that certain variables should be transformed (e.g., log transformation of an interval variable skewed to the right) or that the right variables are not in the model. Unfortunately, journals rarely print residual plots; the reader must rely on the investigators to have reviewed them.

HOW WELL DOES THE MODEL PREDICT OUTCOME?

To assess the power of a linear regression models model in predicting outcome, most investigators report the adjusted R^2. The value of R^2 ranges form 0 to 1; multiplied by 100, R^2 can be thought of as the percentage of the variance in the outcome accounted for by the independent variables. Because R^2 increases in value as additional variables are included in the model, adjusted R^2 charges a penalty for every additional variable included. In a model with a R^2 close to 1, the dependent variables taken together, accurately predict outcome.

For logistic regression models, investigators often report the *Hosmer-Lemeshow goodness-of-fit test*. [25] This statistic compares the estimated to observed likelihood of outcome for groups of subjects. In a well-fitting model, the estimated likelihood will be close to that observed. Readers should be aware that the Hosmer-Lemeshow goodness-of-fit test, along with other available goodness-of-fit statistics, [26] has significant limitations.

Although they exist, goodness-of-fit tests are rarely reported with proportional hazards regression. Instead, some investigators compare estimated to observed time to outcome in tabular form. [27] In a well fitting model, the estimated and observed times to outcome for different groups of subjects will be similar.

Although, goodness-of-fit statistics are an adequate measure of how well an explanatory model predicts outcome, predictive models require a more quantitative measure of their success in predicting outcome. This is commonly done with a logistic regression model by computing the sensitivity, specificity and accuracy of a model's predictions at a particular cut-point. The area under the receiver-operator characteristic (ROC) curves allow assessment of the predictive value of a logistic regression model over a variety of cut-offs of probability of outcome. [28, 29]

IS THE MODEL RELIABLE?

Readers should see if the author has shown that a multivariable is reliable before accepting it at face value. The reliability of a model depends on its purpose. If it is an explanatory model, reliability means that a different set of data would likely yield the same terms in the model with similar coefficients. A reliable predictive model means that it predicts outcomes equally well in other settings or on data other than the ones in which it was developed.

Although, some decrement in performance is acceptable when a model is rerun with new data, a reliable model will perform well with new data. Unfortunately, it is not always possible for investigators to collect additional data. In these situations, investigators may report one of three alternative methods for assessing the reliability of a model: *split-group*, *jackknife*, and *bootstrap*. [1] With split-group validation the investigators divide the data set into two parts; the model is developed on the first dataset and then validated on the second dataset. With a jackknife procedure the investigator sequentially deletes subjects from a data set and repeatedly recomputes the model with each subject missing once. With a bootstrap procedure, the investigators take random samples of subjects from a data set with replacement (meaning that a subject may be chosen more than once). Although none of these methods can be considered definitive, if they closely approximate the original model, readers can have greater confidence in the results.

CONCLUSION

Multivariable analysis is critical to the field of perinatology. When performed and interpreted correctly, these models deepen our understanding of important perinatal outcomes. At the same time, it is important to remember the limitations of multivariable analysis. For example, although it is possible to adjust for known predictors of an outcome we can only adjust for those confounders that we know and have measured. Most importantly, models are only helpful to the extent that the data fit the assumptions of it.

REFERENCES

[1] Katz MH. *Multivariable analysis: A practical guide for clinicians* (third edition). New York: Cambridge University Press, 2011.

[2] Chen KT, Segúu M, Lumey LH, et al. Genital herpes simplex virus infection and perinatal transmission of human immunodeficiency virus. *Obstet Gynecol.* 2005;106:1341-8.

[3] Kimberlin DF, Hauth JC, Owen J, et al. Indicated versus spontaneous preterm delivery: An evaluation of neonatal morbidity among infants weighing ≤1000 grams at birth. *Am J Obstet Gynecol* 1999;180:683-9.

[4] Starr R, Zurawski J, Mahmoud I. Preoperative vaginal preparation with povidone-iodine and the risk of postcesarean endometritis. *Obstet Gynecol.* 2005;105:1024-9.

[5] Geerts L, Odendaal HJ. Severe early onset pre-eclampsia: prognostic value of ultrasound and Doppler assessment. *J Perinatology.* 2007;27: 335-342.

[6] Harrell FE., Jr. *Regression Modeling Strategies: With applications to linear models, logistic regression and survival analysis.* New York: Springer, 2001, p. 4.

[7] Erez O, Robero R, Espinoza J, et al. The change in concentrations of angiogenic and anti-angiogenic factors in maternal plasma between the first and second trimesters in risk assessment for the subsequent development of preeclampsia and small-for-gestational age. *J Matern Fetal Neonatal Med.* 2008;21(5):279-287.

[8] Wy CA, Sajous CH, Loberiza F, Weiss MG. Outcome of infants with a diagnosis of hydrops fetalis in the 1990s. *Am J Perinatol* 1999;16:561-7.

[9] Sperling RS, Shapiro DE, Coombs RW, et al. Maternal viral load, zidovudine treatment, and the risk of transmission of human immunodeficiency virus type 1 from mother to infant. *N Engl J Med.* 1996;335:1621-9.

[10] Phibbs CS, Bronstein JM, Buxton E, Phibbs RH. The effects of patient volume and level of care at the hospital of birth on neonatal mortality. *JAMA.* 1996;276:1054-49.

[11] Peduzzi P, Concato J, Kemper Ed, Holdord TR, Feinstein AR. A simulation study of the number of events per variable in logistic regression analysis. *J Clin Epidemiol.* 1996;49:1373-9.

[12] Peduzzi P, Concato J, Feinstein AR, Holford TR. Importance of events per independent variable in proportional hazards regression analysis II. Accuracy and precision of regression estimates. *J Clin Epidemiol.* 1995;48:1503-10.

[13] Harrell FE, Lee KL, Matchar DB, Reichert TA. Regression models for prognostic prediction: advantages, problems, and suggested solutions. *Cancer Treat Rep.* 1985;69:1071-7.

[14] Greenland S. Modeling and variable selection in epidemiologic analysis. *Am J Public Health.* 1989;79:340-9.

[15] Steyerberg EW, Eijkemans MJ, Habbema JD. Stepwise selection in small data sets: a simulation study of bias in logistic regression analysis. *J Clin Epidemiol.* 1999;52:935-42.

[16] Harrell F, Lee K, Mark D. Multivariable prognostic models: Issues in developing models, evaluating assumptions and adequacy, and measuring and reducing errors. *Statistics in Medicine*. 1996;15:361-87.

[17] Kahn HA, Sempos CT. *Statistical methods in epidemiology*. New York: Oxford University Press, 1989, pp. 193-8.

[18] Lawless JF. *Statistical models and methods for lifetime data*. New York: John Wiley and Sons, 1982, pp. 394-5.

[19] Kalbfleish JD, Prentice RL. *The statistical analysis of failure time data*. New York: John Wiley and Sons, 1980, pp. 89-98.

[20] Kelsey JL, Whittemore AS, Evans AS, Thompson WD. *Methods in observational epidemiology*. New York: Oxford University Press, 1996, pp. 130-4.

[21] Twisk JWR. Applied *Longitudinal Data Analysis for Epidemiology: A Practical Guide*. Cambridge University Press, 2003, pp. 62-92.

[22] Diggle PJ, Heagerty P, Liang K-Y, Zeger SL. *Analysis of Longitudinal Data* (second edn). Oxford: Oxford University Press, 2002, pp 141-189.

[23] Smith GCS, Shah I, Crossley JA, et al. Pregnancy-associated plasma protein A and alpha-fetoprotein and prediction of adverse perinatal outcome. *Obstet Gynecol*. 2006;107:161-6.

[24] Glantz SA, Slinker BK. *Primer of applied regression and analysis of variance*. New York: McGraw-Hill, 1990, pp. 110-80.

[25] Hosmer DW, Lemeshow S. *Applied Logistic Regression*. New York: Wiley, 1989, pp. 187-215.

[26] Hosmer DW, Hosmer T, Le Cessie S, Lemeshow S. A comparison of goodness-of-fit tests for the logistic regression model. *Statistics in Medicine*. 1997;16:965-80.

[27] Colford JM Jr, Tager IB, Hirozawa AM, Lemp GF, Aragon T, Petersen C. Cryptosporidiosis among patients infected with human immunodeficiency virus. Factors related to symptomatic infection and survival. *Am J Epidemiol*. 1996;144:807-16.

[28] Hanley JA, McNeil BJ. The meaning and use of the area under a receiver operating characteristic (ROC) curve. *Radiology*. 1982;143:29-36.

[29] Hsiao JK, Bartko JJ, Potter WZ. Diagnosing diagnoses. Receiver operating characteristic methods and psychiatry. *Arch Gen Psychiatry*. 1989;46:664-7.

In: Handbook of Methodological Concepts in Perinatal Medicine   ISBN: 978-1-62081-252-5
Editor: Eyal Sheiner   © 2013 Nova Science Publishers, Inc.

Chapter 8

PRACTICAL GUIDE FOR DATA ANALYSIS OF PERINATAL EPIDEMIOLOGY BY SPSS®

Amalia Levy

Epidemiology and Health Services Evaluation Department, Faculty of Health Sciences,
Ben-Gurion University of the Negev, Israel

INTRODUCTION

As researchers, we usually start with scientific questions that lead us to our study hypotheses; we then plan and perform the study by collecting data from a subset of the population, our sample. Next, we analyze the collected data while using statistical tools to reach conclusions regarding the population.

This chapter gives a brief overview of the principles of data analysis within perinatal epidemiology studies; however, this will not include all of the important stages of a study. In addition, the examples shown in this chapter are the most common statistical tests in perinatal epidemiology only. In order to learn the most when reading this chapter, one needs a basic knowledge of statistics and SPSS®.

THE STEPS OF DATA ANALYSIS

A typical data analysis includes three major steps:

1) Univariable analysis, which comprises mainly descriptive statistics and graphs describing the characteristics of the participants of a study. In this step, we begin by looking at the distribution of the variables as well as trying to discover and correct data errors that may occur. We also check whether our variable distributions are normal. Checking normality can be done by looking at the graphs, central tendency (mean, median, and mode), and the values of skewness and kurtosis, or by applying appropriate statistical tests.

2) Bivariable analysis tests the relationship between two variables or the differences between groups of people. For example, linear relationship is measured by a correlation, but the outcome can also be predicted by a single predictor using simple regression. Comparison of the means of two independent groups can be performed by student t-tests.

3) Multivariable analysis predicts an outcome from several predictor variables, or examines one variable in relation to the outcome variable while adjusting for all other variables (multiple regressions).

CHOOSING THE SUITABLE STATISTICAL TEST

The principles of choosing the suitable statistical test for the three major steps mentioned above are provided in all statistics books.

Following are the principles, summarized very briefly:

1) The scientific study questions or the study hypothesis (relation between the variables, comparing groups or prediction).

2) The study type or outline (comparison between or within groups and the number of comparisons).

3) The variable type, such as continuous or categorical.

4) The variable distribution—whether a sample originates from a normally distributed population.

5) Sample size or number of observations in the compared groups, e.g., 30 or more observations per group.

WORKING WITH SPSS FOR WINDOWS®

SPSS includes three types of files: the SPSS data editor, syntax, and the viewer (the output) [1–3].

The SPSS data editor is the file including all the study data that can be either imported from other types of files or entered directly to the SPSS file. The data editor has two views: the "data view" and the "variable view".

The data view is constructed of columns and rows: each column is a variable and each row is a participant in the study; as a result, each cell is a variable's value for a certain person in the study (Figure 1).

The second view is the variable view, which includes the variables' definitions, such as name, type, label, missing values, and measure (Figure 2).

We can shift from data view to variable view by clicking on the tabs shown in the bottom left side of the screen (see arrow in Figure 3).

	sno	gender	race	in_hosp_date	dis_date	i_b_date	m_b_date	ap1
1	1	2	1	02-JAN-2005	10-JAN-2005	04-JAN-2005	02-NOV-1972	8
2	2	1	2	09-JAN-2005	13-JAN-2005	09-JAN-2005	02-APR-1975	1
3	3	1	1	30-JAN-2005	01-FEB-2005	30-JAN-2005	16-MAY-1967	9
4	5	1	1	19-MAR-2005	24-MAR-2005	20-MAR-2005	24-FEB-1966	9
5	6	2	1	20-MAR-2005	25-MAR-2005	21-MAR-2005	01-JAN-1970	9
6	7	2	1	02-AUG-2005	07-AUG-2005	03-AUG-2005	21-OCT-1977	9
7	8	2	1	30-MAY-2005	04-JUN-2005	30-MAY-2005	26-JUN-1975	9
8	9	2	2	20-DEC-2005	24-DEC-2005	20-DEC-2005	02-JUN-1976	9
9	10	1	1	18-JUL-2005	25-JUL-2005	19-JUL-2005	08-DEC-1974	9
10	11	1	1	27-NOV-2005	28-NOV-2005	28-NOV-2005	15-AUG-1980	.
11	12	1	1	22-AUG-2005	28-AUG-2005	22-AUG-2005	07-FEB-1971	9
12	13	1	2	02-FEB-2005	06-FEB-2005	03-FEB-2005	12-APR-1976	9
13	14	1	1	07-FEB-2005	.	07-FEB-2005	22-JUL-1973	.
14	15	2	1	26-APR-2005	29-APR-2005	26-APR-2005	31-JAN-1969	9
15	16	1	1	04-NOV-2005	06-NOV-2005	04-NOV-2005	20-APR-1974	9
16	17	2	1	03-MAY-2005	06-MAY-2005	04-MAY-2005	26-JUN-1974	9
17	18	1	1	03-JAN-2005	05-JAN-2005	04-JAN-2005	20-MAY-1965	9
18	19	1	2	13-APR-2005	20-APR-2005	18-APR-2005	31-JUL-1974	9
19	20	2	1	25-JAN-2005	27-JAN-2005	25-JAN-2005	15-JUL-1978	9
20	21	1	1	16-JAN-2005	18-JAN-2005	16-JAN-2005	14-OCT-1975	9
21	22	1	2	09-MAR-2005	12-MAR-2005	10-MAR-2005	16-AUG-1983	9
22	23	2	1	14-NOV-2005	18-NOV-2005	15-NOV-2005	25-MAY-1971	9
23	24	1	1	20-NOV-2005	27-NOV-2005	23-NOV-2005	27-JAN-1972	.
24	25	1	1	20-NOV-2005	23-NOV-2005	21-NOV-2005	01-JUN-1971	9
25	26	1	1	30-JAN-2005	01-FEB-2005	30-JAN-2005	26-JAN-1973	9
26	27	1	1	03-JAN-2005	06-JAN-2005	04-JAN-2005	19-JUN-1972	9
27	28	1	2	22-NOV-2005	24-NOV-2005	22-NOV-2005	07-NOV-1981	9

Figure 1. The Data View of the SPSS Data Editor.

	Name	Type	Width	Decimals	Label	Values	Missing	Columns	Align	Measure
1	sno	Numeric	4	0	Serial number	None	None	8	Center	Nominal
2	gender	Numeric	1	0	Gender	{1, Male}...	None	8	Center	Nominal
3	race	Numeric	1	0	Race	{1, Caucasian }...	None	10	Center	Nominal
4	in_hosp_da	Date	11	0	Mother's hospitalization date	None	None	11	Center	Scale
5	dis_date	Date	11	0	Discharge date from hospitalization	None	None	11	Center	Scale
6	i_b_date	Date	11	0	Infant's birth date	None	None	11	Center	Scale
7	m_b_date	Date	11	0	Mother's birth date	None	None	11	Center	Scale
8	ap1	Numeric	8	0	Apgar at 1st minute	None	None	8	Center	Ordinal
9	ap5	Numeric	8	0	Apgar at 5th minute	None	None	8	Center	Ordinal
10	birth_weigh	Numeric	8	0	Birth-weight (in grams)	None	None	8	Center	Scale
11	ges_days	Numeric	8	0	Gestational age (in days)	None	None	8	Center	Scale
12	s_a_l_ges_	Numeric	8	0	SGA/AGA/LGA	{1, SGA}...	None	15	Right	Ordinal
13	APD	Numeric	8	0	Ante Partum Death	{0, No }...	None	8	Center	Nominal
14	IPD	Numeric	8	0	Intra Partum Death	{0, No }...	None	8	Center	Nominal
15	PPD	Numeric	8	0	Post Partum Death	{0, No }...	None	10	Center	Nominal
16	death_date	Date	11	0	Date of infant's death	None	None	10	Center	Scale
17	preg_num	Numeric	8	0	Number of pregnancies	None	None	8	Center	Scale
18	birth_num	Numeric	8	0	Number of births	None	None	8	Center	Scale
19	adver_obs_	Numeric	8	0	Adverse obstetric history	{0, No }...	None	11	Center	Nominal
20	rec_abor	Numeric	8	0	Recurrent abortions	{0, No }...	None	8	Center	Nominal
21	pre_prema	Numeric	8	0	Previous premature labor	{0, No }...	None	13	Center	Nominal
22	infert_treat	Numeric	8	0	Infertility treatments	{0, No }...	None	8	Center	Nominal
23	poly	Numeric	8	0	Polyhydramnios	{0, No }...	None	8	Center	Nominal
24	oligo	Numeric	8	0	Oligohydramnios	{0, No }...	None	8	Center	Nominal
25	amniocynt	Numeric	8	0	Amniocyntesis	{0, No }...	None	12	Center	Nominal
26	PROM	Numeric	8	0	Premature rapture of membranes	{0, No }...	None	8	Center	Nominal

Figure 2. The Variable View of the SPSS Data Editor.

10	11	1	1	27-NOV-2005	28-NOV-2005
11	12	1	1	22-AUG-2005	28-AUG-2005
12	13	1	2	02-FEB-2005	06-FEB-2005
13	14	1	1	07-FEB-2005	
14	15	2	1	26-APR-2005	29-APR-2005
15	16	1	1	04-NOV-2005	06-NOV-2005
16	17	2	1	03-MAY-2005	06-MAY-2005
17	18	1	1	03-JAN-2005	05-JAN-2005
18	19	1	2	13-APR-2005	20-APR-2005
19	20	2	1	25-JAN-2005	27-JAN-2005
20	21	1	1	16-JAN-2005	18-JAN-2005
21	22	1	2	09-MAR-2005	12-MAR-2005
22	23	2	1	14-NOV-2005	18-NOV-2005
23	24	1	1	20-NOV-2005	27-NOV-2005
24	25	1	1	20-NOV-2005	23-NOV-2005
25	26	1	1	30-JAN-2005	01-FEB-2005
26	27	1	1	03-JAN-2005	06-JAN-2005
27	28		2	22-NOV-2005	24-NOV-2005
28	29	2	2	23-FEB-2005	24-FEB-2005
29	30	2	1	21-MAR-2005	23-MAR-2005
30	31	2	2	25-AUG-2005	28-AUG-2005
31	32	2	2	14-MAY-2005	16-MAY-2005
32		2	2	14-AUG-2005	16-AUG-2005
33	34	2	2	19-NOV-2005	21-NOV-2005

◄ ► \ Data View λ Variable View /

Figure 3. Shifting between Data View and Variable View.

The SPSS syntax is the file with the commands (as transformations) and procedures (the statistical analyses) [1–3]. We will create commands and procedures by using the SPSS dialog box. While using the dialog box, we can choose one of two options "OK" or "Paste". The recommended way of working is by clicking on the Paste tab rather than the OK tab because it creates documentation of written commands and procedures while OK does not. This is very important, especially when working on transformation variables. An example of syntax created automatically after choosing to work with the Paste option is shown in Figure 4.

The viewer is the SPSS output file [1–3]. In this file we will find the results after running the syntax file (see arrow in Figure 4). All commands and procedures will be performed on the data file, creating an output file. The next paragraphs will include examples of output files and further explanations.

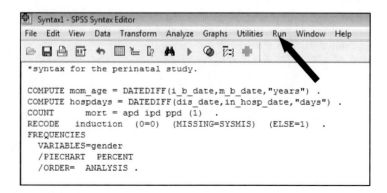

Figure 4. Example of a Syntax File.

Perinatal Data Analysis

Let us assume that we have a data file of a small obstetric department that includes information about 1200 mothers who gave birth during 2005. The data file includes variables such as demographic characteristics, chronic diseases, obstetric history, and information about the labor as well as the newborn (Addendum 1 includes the list of the study variables). In order to simplify the data analysis process, the data file consists of singleton births only.

Addendum 1. The Study Variables List

Variable name	Variable label	Variable values
gender	Gender	1 Male, 2 Female
race	Race	1 Caucasian, 2 Afro-American
in_hosp_date	Mother's hospitalization date	
dis_date	Discharge date from hospitalization	
i_b_date	Infant's birth date	
m_b_date	Mother's birth date	
ap1	Apgar at 1st minute	
ap5	Apgar at 5th minute	
birth_weight	Birth-weight (in grams)	
ges_days	Gestational age (in days)	
s_a_l_ges_age	SGA/AGA/LGA	1 SGA, 2 AGA, 3 LGA
APD	Ante Partum Death	0 No, 1 Yes
IPD	Intra Partum Death	0 No, 1 Yes
PPD	Post Partum Death	0 No, 1 Yes
preg_num	Number of pregnancies	
birth_num	Number of births	
infert_treat	Infertility treatments	0 No, 1 Yes
poly	Polyhydramnios	0 No, 1 Yes
oligo	Oligohydramnios	0 No, 1 Yes
PROM	Premature rapture of membranes	0 No, 1 Yes
Cervical_incomp	Cervical incompetence	0 No, 1 Yes
placental_abru	Placental abruption	0 No, 1 Yes
placenta_previa	Placenta previa	0 No, 1 Yes
mal_presnt	Mal-presentation	0 No, 1 Yes
Malfor	Congenital malformations	0 No, 1 Yes
iugr	Intra uterine growth restriction	0 No, 1 Yes
fet_dist	Fetal distress	0 No, 1 Yes
miconium	Meconium stained amniotic fluid	0 No, 1 Yes
induction	Labor induction	0 No, 1 Yes
epidural	Epidural anesthesia	0 No, 1 Yes
general_anes	General anesthesia	0 No, 1 Yes
spontaneous_del	Spontaneous delivery	0 No, 1 Yes
cd	Caesarian delivery	0 No, 1 Yes
vacuum	Vacuum delivery	0 No, 1 Yes
post_pa_hemo	Post partum hemorrhage	0 No, 1 Yes
ret_placenta	Retained placenta	0 No, 1 Yes
Mild_pree	Mild preeclampsia	0 No, 1 Yes
severe_pree	Severe preeclampsia	0 No, 1 Yes
chr_htn	Chronic hypertension	0 No, 1 Yes
get_dm	Gestational diabetes mellitus	0 No, 1 Yes
dm	Diabetes Mellitus	0 No, 1 Yes
hemoglobin1	Maternal hemoglobin before delivery (g/dL)	0 No, 1 Yes
hemoglobin2	Maternal hemoglobin after delivery (g/dL)	0 No, 1 Yes

1. Descriptive Statistics

First of all, we would like to conduct a univariable analysis using mainly descriptive statistics [4]. The most common way is by using the "Frequencies" procedure. For example, we can present the gender distribution of the study's infants using a table and a chart [1–3].

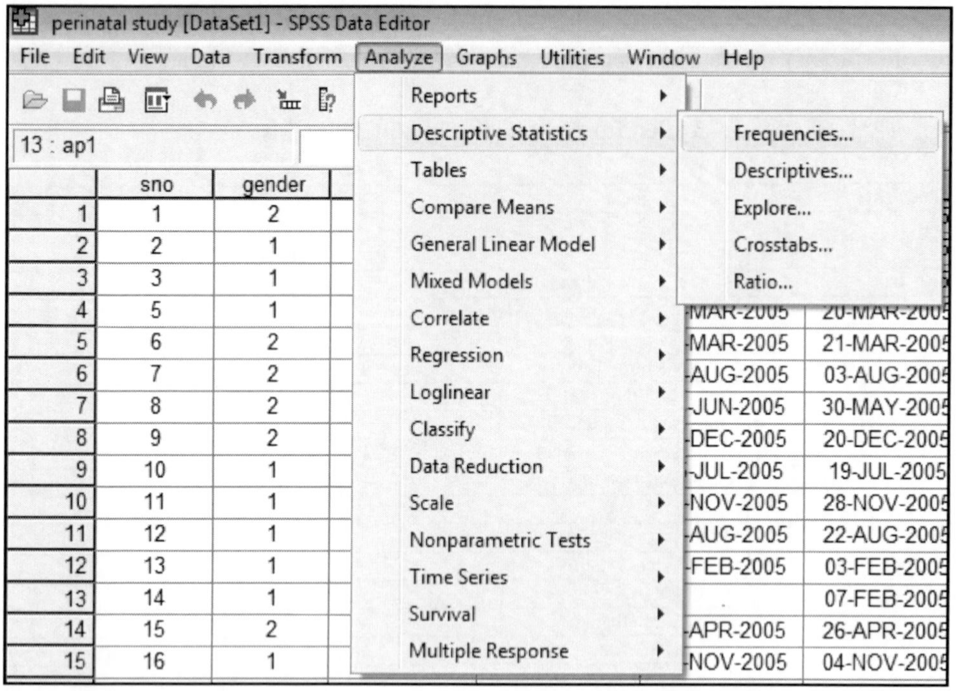

Figure 5. Descriptive Statistics of the Frequencies Procedure.

After opening the data file we should click on *Analyze* > *Descriptive statistics*>*Frequencies* (Figure 5). Clicking on "Frequencies" will open the window shown in Figure 6. Now we choose the variables we would like to include in the procedure from the list on the left, simply by clicking on the variable name (Figure 6, 1) and then transferring it to the right window using the arrow button (Figure 6, 2). In all SPSS procedures the list on the left, presenting all the study variables, will appear in the same order as in the data file.

Now we can add the appropriate chart according to the descriptive statistics rules. In the Frequencies window we have to click on *Frequencie s> Charts > Pie charts* (Figure 7). Now we can click on "Continue" and return to the main window. Clicking on Paste will automatically open a syntax file with the following text:

- FREQUENCIES
- VARIABLES=gender
- /PIECHART PERCENT
- /ORDER=ANALYSIS.

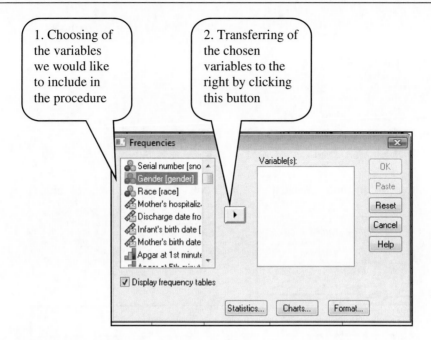

Figure 6. The Frequencies Procedure.

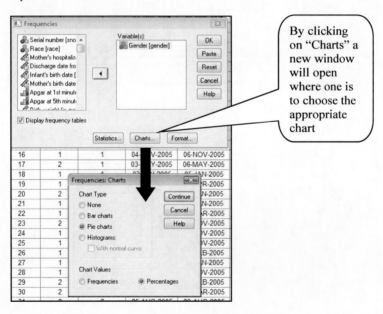

Figure 7. Adding a Chart to the Frequencies Procedure.

After running the Frequencies procedure, we will receive an output file that will look as shown in Figure 8.

Frequencies

In the case of a continuous variable, such as birth weight, we can add statistics such as mean, median, mode, and standard deviation:

- Analyze> Descriptive statistics> Frequencies> Statistics>mean, median…

And the syntax will be:

- FREQUENCIES
- VARIABLES=birth_weight
- /STATISTICS=STDDEV MEAN MEDIAN MODE
- /ORDER=ANALYSIS.

The output will include the statistics table followed by the frequencies table (Figure 9).

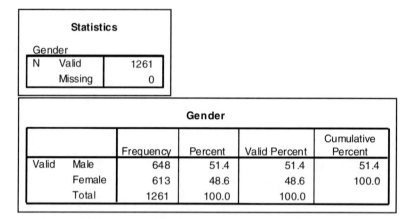

Statistics

Gender

N	Valid	1261
	Missing	0

Gender

		Frequency	Percent	Valid Percent	Cumulative Percent
Valid	Male	648	51.4	51.4	51.4
	Female	613	48.6	48.6	100.0
	Total	1261	100.0	100.0	

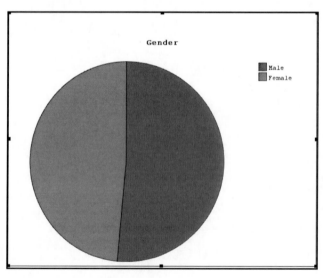

Figure 8. The Output File Including the Frequencies Table and the Chart.

2. Transformations

Transformation is the creation of new variables according to the study hypothesis [1-3. For example, we calculate the mother's age (in years) at time of delivery, or the hospitalization duration (in days). In addition, we can create new variables by recoding the original variables, for instance, the variable of low Apgar scores (<7) at 1 minute and 5 minutes is created through the recoding of the original Apgar scores.

Another example of such transformation can be done when recoding the original birth weight variable to a low birth weight variable (<2500 g). Furthermore, we can construct a new variable, such as infant mortality, according to the APD, IPD, and PPD values, which had all been originally included in the data file.

Statistics

Birth-weight (in grams)

N	Valid	1261
	Missing	0
Mean		3157.27
Median		3215.00
Mode		3095
Std. Deviation		571.249

Birth-weight (in grams)

		Frequency	Percent	Valid Percent	Cumulative Percent
Valid	350	1	.1	.1	.1
	476	1	.1	.1	.2
	532	1	.1	.1	.2
	550	1	.1	.1	.3
	675	1	.1	.1	.4
	780	1	.1	.1	.5
	793	1	.1	.1	.6
	836	1	.1	.1	.6
	886	1	.1	.1	.7
	978	1	.1	.1	.8
	988	1	.1	.1	.9
	1008	1	.1	.1	1.0
	1158	1	.1	.1	1.0
	1160	1	.1	.1	1.1

Figure 9. The Output File Including the Statistics and the Frequencies Tables.

Calculating the Mother's Age

The mother's age variable can be calculated by clicking the following [1-3].

- Transform> Compute…

The window shown in Figure 10 will then open. First, we type the "Target Variable" (Figure 10, 1)—for example, "mom_age"; next we choose the "Function group" needed (Figure 10, 2), which in this case of calculating the mother's age it is "Date Arithmetic"; afterwards we choose the function "Datediff" (Figure 10, 3) that calculates the time difference between any two dates, using any time units (years, months, or days…).

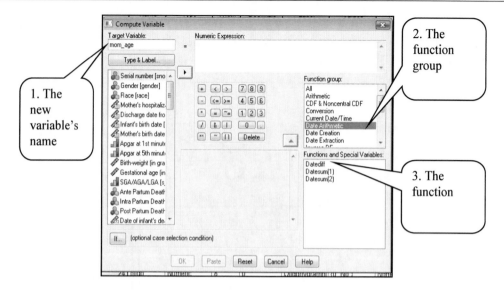

Figure 10. Computing Time Interval from two Date Variables.

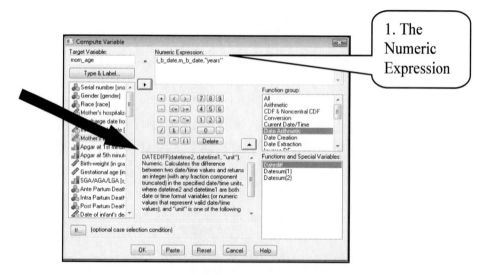

Figure 11. The Numeric Expression of the New Variable.

After choosing "Datediff", we insert the "Numeric Expression" (Figure 11, 1). The pattern of the Numeric Expression should be as follows: datetime2, datetime1, "unit" (see arrow in Figure 11). For example, when calculating the mother's age (in years) at the time of giving birth, the pattern of the Numeric Expression is: infant's birth date, mother's birth date, "years" (Figure 11, 1).

Finally, we click the Paste button, which will result the following syntax:

- COMPUTE mom_age = DATEDIFF(i_b_date,m_b_date,"years").

In the same way we can create a new variable of hospitalization duration (in days) by calculating the time difference between the mother's discharge date from the hospital and the mother's hospitalization date. In this case, the syntax is:

- COMPUTE hospdays=DATEDIFF(dis_date,in_hosp_date,"days".

Creating a New Variable – Infant Mortality

Sometime we create a new variable by summarizing other variables. For example, our data include three variables of infant mortality: APD, IPD, and PPD (Ante-Partum Death, Intra-Partum Death, and Post-Partum Death, respectively). After examining each of the original variables separately, we can create a new variable of infant mortality. Logically, if the answer to one of the original variables is "yes", the result of the new infant mortality variable would also be "yes". If our data have no errors, then only one variable can be "yes". We can count the number of positive answers and the total will represent the value of infant mortality.

In "Transform" click the following [1-3]:

- Transform > Count...

As shown in the window in Figure 12, we type the name of the target variable – for instance, "infant_mortality" (Figure 12, 1); then we define the variables that constitute the new variable (APD, IPD, and PPD) as depicted in Figure 12, number 2.

Next, we click on "Define Values" (see arrow in Figure 12) in order to define the values that are going to be counted, for instance in the example shown below, it is "1" (see arrow in Figure 13).

We can also define ranges of values if needed, as shown in Figure 13. After clicking on the "Continue" button, you then click on Paste, which will result the following syntax:

- COUNT infant_mortality=APD IPD PPD (1)

When running this syntax, the new variable will be created in the data file.

3. Bivariable Analysis

Bivariable analysis is the testing of the relationship between two variables or the differences between groups of the study participants. [4, 5] Two or more groups can be compared, for example, by the comparison of the variables' means. The decision to perform comparison of means should be done according to the statistical rules mentioned in the beginning of this chapter. For example, we can compare the birth weight of infants born with or without congenital malformations. When comparing between just two groups, the t-test is preferred. In the case of three or more groups, the One-Way ANOVA test is to be performed.

In order to compare the variables' means we do the following: [1–3]

- Analyze> Compare Means>Independent-Samples T-Test...

As shown in Figure 14, you can choose from all the procedures for comparing means, including the Independent-Samples T-Test, the paired-samples T-Test, as well as the One-Way ANOVA.

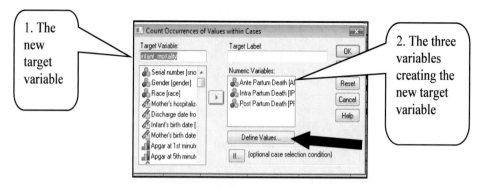

Figure 12. Creating New Variable by Counting Values.

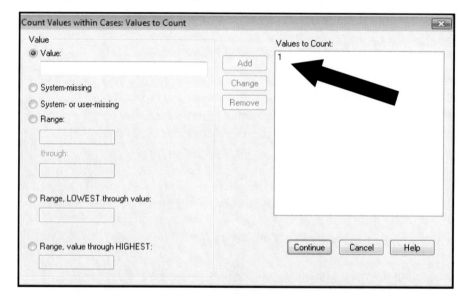

Figure 13. Defining the Values to be counted.

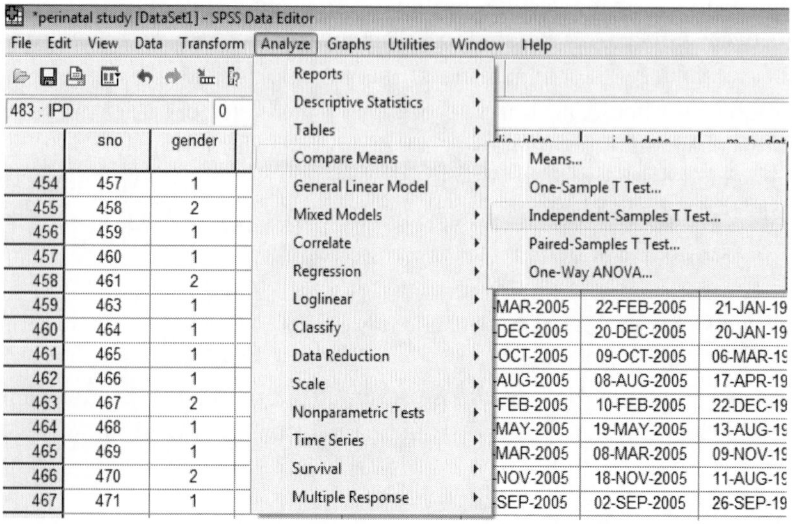

Figure 14. Comparison of Means Procedures.

When clicking on "Independent-Samples T-Test..." the window shown in Figure 15 will open. There, we will define the tested or the dependent variable (Figure 15, 1), in addition to the grouping variable or the independent variable (Figure 15, 2).

Again, click on Paste, which will result the following syntax:

Once the syntax is running, an output file will be created. An output file looks as depicted in Figure 16; it includes the descriptive statistics table and the t-test table.

From the descriptive statistics table we can see that newborns with congenital malformations have a lower mean birth weight (2903.68 g ± 849.47 g) compared to newborns without congenital malformations (3183.21 g ± 528.43 g) (Figure 16, 1). Examining the second table detects that "Leven's Test for Equality of Variances" is statistically significant (p < 0.001) (Figure 16, 2), meaning that we cannot assume equal variances (we reject the null hypothesis of equality of variances). As a result, we look at the second row of the t-test values. The result of the birth weight comparison according to the t-test procedure is statistically significant (p = 0.001) (Figure 16, 3).

The reported results should be written as follows: the mean birth weight of newborns with congenital malformations was found to be lower than newborns without congenital malformations (2903.68 ± 849.47 g and 3183.21 ± 528.43 g, respectively) (p = 0.001).

- T-TEST
- GROUPS=malformations(0 1)
- /MISSING=ANALYSIS
- /VARIABLES=birth_weight
- /CRITERIA=CI(.95).

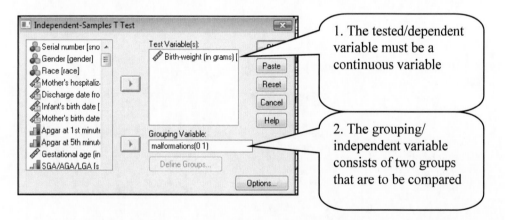

Figure 15. Defining the Test Variable and the Grouping Variable of the Independent Sample t-test Procedure.

Occasionally, during the course of a study, certain observations are measured several times. The simplest situation is when we have a set of two repeated measurements; for example, in our study there are two hemoglobin test results, before and after delivery; therefore, we can examine the hypothesis of a decrease in hemoglobin level at the time of labor. In such a situation, the suitable statistical test is paired-samples t-test. Unlike in the previous example, we have two continuous variables that are measured at two different times during the study, instead of the comparison of the means of two groups.

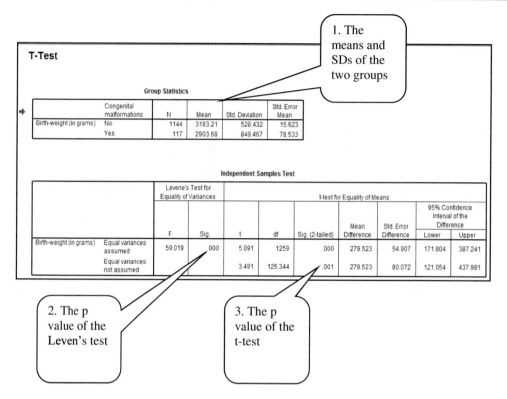

Figure 16. The Independent-Samples t-test Output.

In order to perform a comparison of two paired means, we will do the following: [1–3]

- Analyze> Compare Means> paired-samples T-Test

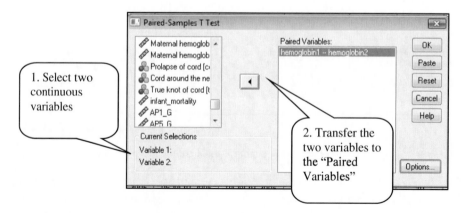

Figure 17. The Paired-samples t-test Procedure.

The screen shown in Figure 17 will appear. Only when choosing both of the variables (Variable 1, Variable 2) (Figure 17, 1), can we transfer the two to the "Paired Variables" on the right (Figure 17, 2).

- T-TEST
- PAIRS=hemoglobin1 WITH hemoglobin2 (PAIRED)
- /CRITERIA=CI(.95)
- /MISSING=ANALYSIS.
-

Once the syntax above has been run, the output shown in Figure 18 will be created.

T-Test

The output of the paired-samples t-test (Figure 18) consists of 3 tables: the first table is the descriptive statistics of the two variables – the mean and the standard deviation of the hemoglobin levels, before and after delivery. Note how the mean of the hemoglobin after delivery is lower than the hemoglobin mean before delivery. The middle table presents the correlation between the variables, which were found to be statistically significant. The last table is the result of the paired t-test, which shows that the difference between the hemoglobin means, before and after delivery, is statistically significant ($p < 0.001$).

Bivariable analysis can also compare the proportions/rates of two categorical variables. [4, 5] For example, we would like to compare the proportions of cesarean deliveries in newborns with congenital malformations to newborns without ongenital malformations. In this example, the two variables are referred to as "dichotomous variables", where these variables have only two groups; therefore, the suitable statistical tests are the chi-square test, or the Fisher's exact test, both of which examine the differences in qualitative variables.

Paired Samples Statistics		Mean	N	Std. Deviation	Std. Error Mean
Pair 1	Maternal hemoglobin before delivery (gr/dl)	12.704	766	1.9757	.0714
	Maternal hemoglobin after delivery (gr/dl)	10.991	766	1.4630	.0529

Paired Samples Correlations		N	Correlation	Sig.
Pair 1	Maternal hemoglobin before delivery (gr/dl) & Maternal hemoglobin after delivery (gr/dl)	766	.101	.005

Paired Samples Test		Paired Differences					t	df	Sig. (2-tailed)
		Mean	Std. Deviation	Std. Error Mean	95% Confidence Interval of the Difference				
					Lower	Upper			
Pair 1	Maternal hemoglobin before delivery (gr/dl) - Maternal hemoglobin after delivery (gr/dl)	1.7128	2.3372	.0844	1.5470	1.8785	20.283	765	.000

Figure 18. The Paired-samples t-test Output.

In order to perform the comparison above, do the following: [1–3]

• Analyze>Descriptive Statistics >Crosstabs…

The screen shown in Figure 19 will appear.

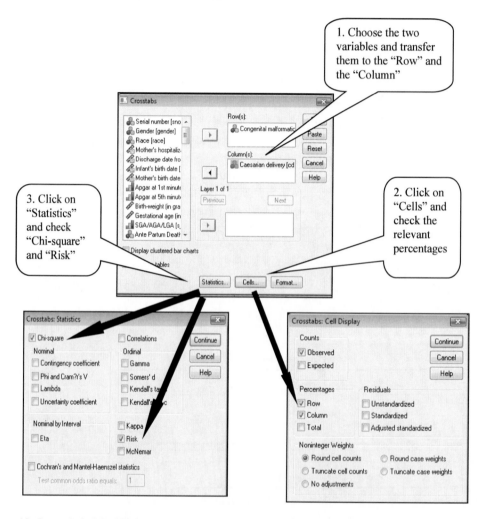

Figure 19. Crosstabulation, Chi-Square Test, and Risk Estimate Procedure.

First choose the variables for the "Crosstabs" procedure (congenital malformations and cesarean delivery), then transfer them to the "Row" and "Column" (Figure 19, 1). After clicking on the "cells" button, check the relevant percentages, such as the percentage of the rows or of the columns (Figure 19, 2). The statistical tests can be added after clicking on "statistics" and checking "Chi-square" and "Risk" (Figure 19, 3).

Once the syntax below is running, an output file is created (Figure 20):

• CROSSTABS
• /TABLES=malformations BY cd
• /FORMAT=AVALUE TABLES

- /STATISTIC=CHISQ RISK
- /CELLS=COUNT ROW COLUMN
- /COUNT ROUND CELL
-

Congenital Malformations * Caesarian Delivery

In some studies the sample size is not big enough; therefore, the table will have over 20% of expected count with values less than 5. In such a case, the Fisher's exact test is the most suitable test. For example, if we compare the proportions of perinatal mortality by congenital malformations, we will obtain the tables shown in Figure 21. We can see that the rate of mortality is 1.0% among infants without malformations, while the rate is 11.1% among infants with malformations.

In the second table (Figure 21) we notice that the Fisher's exact test p value should be used, and not the p value of Pearson's chi-square test.

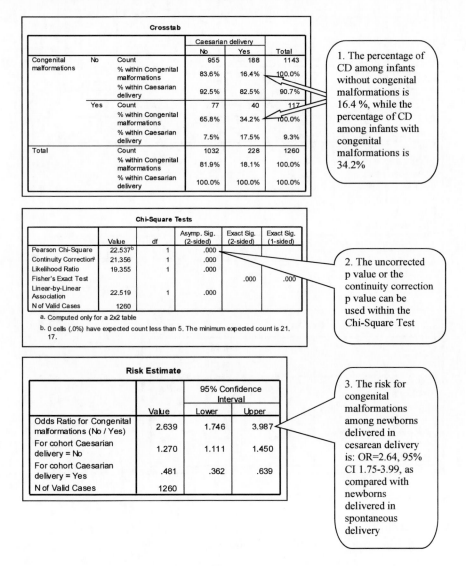

Figure 20. Crosstabulation, Chi Square Test, and Risk Estimate Output.

The last table (Figure 21) presents the risk of mortality, which is OR=12.87, 95% CI 5.63–29.46, and is a measurement of the strength of the association between the presence of a factor and the occurrence of an event. If the confidence interval for the statistic includes a value of 1, one cannot assume that the factor is associated with the event. The odds ratio (OR) can be used as an estimate of relative risk when the occurrence of the factor is rare. [5–8]

Congenital malformations * infant_mortality Crosstabulation

			infant_mortality		Total
			.00	1.00	
Congenital malformations	No	Count	1133	11	1144
		% within Congenital malformations	99.0%	1.0%	100.0%
		% within infant_mortality	91.6%	45.8%	90.7%
	Yes	Count	104	13	117
		% within Congenital malformations	88.9%	11.1%	100.0%
		% within infant_mortality	8.4%	54.2%	9.3%
Total		Count	1237	24	1261
		% within Congenital malformations	98.1%	1.9%	100.0%
		% within infant_mortality	100.0%	100.0%	100.0%

Chi-Square Tests

	Value	df	Asymp. Sig. (2-sided)	Exact Sig. (2-sided)	Exact Sig. (1-sided)
Pearson Chi-Square	58.565[b]	1	.000		
Continuity Correction[a]	53.255	1	.000		
Likelihood Ratio	32.000	1	.000		
Fisher's Exact Test				.000	.000
Linear-by-Linear Association	58.519	1	.000		
N of Valid Cases	1261				

a. Computed only for a 2x2 table

b. 1 cells (25.0%) have expected count less than 5. The minimum expected count is 2.23.

Risk Estimate

	Value	95% Confidence Interval	
		Lower	Upper
Odds Ratio for Congenital malformations (No / Yes)	12.875	5.627	29.458
For cohort infant_mortality = .00	1.114	1.045	1.188
For cohort infant_mortality = 1.00	.087	.040	.189
N of Valid Cases	1261		

Figure 21. Crosstabulation, Fisher's Exact Test, and Risk Estimate Output.

- CROSSTABS
- /TABLES=malformations BY infant_mortality
- /FORMAT= AVALUE TABLES

- /STATISTIC=CHISQ
- /CELLS=COUNT ROW COLUMN
- /COUNT ROUND CELL

Once the syntax above is running, the output file in Figure 21 will be created.

lbw * Congenital malformations Crosstabulation

			Congenital malformations		Total
			No	Yes	
lbw	.00	Count	1043	86	1129
		% within lbw	92.4%	7.6%	100.0%
		% within Congenital malformations	91.2%	73.5%	89.5%
	1.00	Count	101	31	132
		% within lbw	76.5%	23.5%	100.0%
		% within Congenital malformations	8.8%	26.5%	10.5%
Total		Count	1144	117	1261
		% within lbw	90.7%	9.3%	100.0%
		% within Congenital malformations	100.0%	100.0%	100.0%

Chi-Square Tests

	Value	df	Asymp. Sig. (2-sided)	Exact Sig. (2-sided)	Exact Sig. (1-sided)
Pearson Chi-Square	35.350[b]	1	.000		
Continuity Correction[a]	33.490	1	.000		
Likelihood Ratio	27.094	1	.000		
Fisher's Exact Test				.000	.000
Linear-by-Linear Association	35.322	1	.000		
N of Valid Cases	1261				

a. Computed only for a 2x2 table

b. 0 cells (.0%) have expected count less than 5. The minimum expected count is 12.25.

Risk Estimate

	Value	95% Confidence Interval	
		Lower	Upper
Odds Ratio for lbw (.00 / 1.00)	3.722	2.353	5.888
For cohort Congenital malformations = No	1.207	1.097	1.329
For cohort Congenital malformations = Yes	.324	.224	.469
N of Valid Cases	1261		

Figure 22. Crosstabulation and Risk Estimate Output.

Crosstabs

4. Multivariable Analysis

The reasons, ways of performing, and interpretations of multivariable analysis are all included in statistics books dealing generally with medical research [9, 10] and particularly perinatology [11]. There are four major reasons for performing multivariable analysis, all of which are detailed in the chapter "The importance of multivariable analysis for conducting and evaluating research in perinatology" in this book.

Stratification Using Mantel-Haenszel Procedure

One of the reasons for conducting stratified analysis is to determine the unique contributions of a single variable on a single outcome while holding other variables constant, thereby eliminating confounding [5–8, 11]. For example, in the bivariable analysis we found that congenital malformations are a significant risk factor for low birth weight (LBW). As seen in Figure 22, the risk for LBW of infants with congenital malformations is 3.72-fold that of infants with normal birth weight (95% CI 2.35–5.89, p < 0.001).

lbw * preterm37 Crosstabulation

			preterm37 .00	preterm37 1.00	Total
lbw	.00	Count	1098	29	1127
		% within lbw	97.4%	2.6%	100.0%
		% within preterm37	95.6%	26.4%	89.5%
	1.00	Count	51	81	132
		% within lbw	38.6%	61.4%	100.0%
		% within preterm37	4.4%	73.6%	10.5%
Total		Count	1149	110	1259
		% within lbw	91.3%	8.7%	100.0%
		% within preterm37	100.0%	100.0%	100.0%

Chi-Square Tests

	Value	df	Asymp. Sig. (2-sided)	Exact Sig. (2-sided)	Exact Sig. (1-sided)
Pearson Chi-Square	512.182[b]	1	.000		
Continuity Correction[a]	504.835	1	.000		
Likelihood Ratio	300.726	1	.000		
Fisher's Exact Test				.000	.000
Linear-by-Linear Association	511.775	1	.000		
N of Valid Cases	1259				

a. Computed only for a 2x2 table

b. 0 cells (.0%) have expected count less than 5. The minimum expected count is 11.53.

Risk Estimate

	Value	95% Confidence Interval Lower	95% Confidence Interval Upper
Odds Ratio for lbw (.00 / 1.00)	60.134	36.159	100.004
For cohort preterm37 = .00	2.522	2.033	3.127
For cohort preterm37 = 1.00	.042	.029	.062
N of Valid Cases	1259		

Figure 23. Crosstabulation and Risk Estimate Output.

As we know, one of the important risk factors for LBW is gestational age. The risk for LBW of infants born in preterm delivery is significantly greater than in infants born in term delivery. The results shown in Figure 23 are based on the definition of preterm delivery of < 37 weeks of gestational age. These results show that the risk is OR=60.13-fold (95% CI 36.16–100.00, p < 0.001).

Since there is an association between congenital malformation and gestational age, the possibility that gestational age may be a confounder should be tested (few epidemiology textbooks can give you further explanations for the concept of confounding) [5–8].

In order to resolve this question, one of the well-known adjustment procedures can be performed, for example, the Mantel-Haenszel procedure [5–8]. This procedure is designed to test the independence between a dichotomous factor variable and a dichotomous response variable, conditional upon covariate patterns defined by one or more layer (control) variable.

We will use the same Crosstabs procedure, adding the 3rd variable – preterm delivery, which is the layer variable (Figure 24, 1) [1–3]. Next, we will click on "statistics" and check the Mantel-Haenszel statistic (Figure 24, 2).

Once the following syntax is running, the output file shown in Figure 25A will be created.

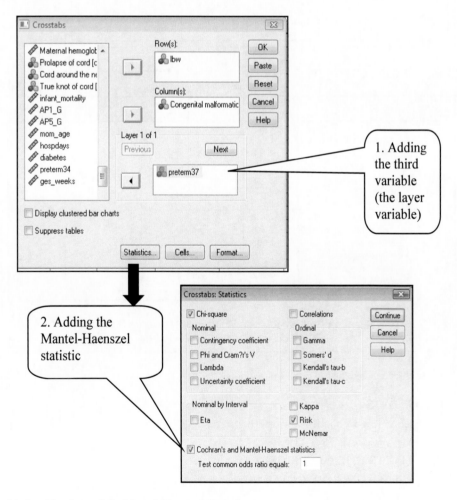

Figure 24. Stratification and the Mantel-Haenszel Procedure.

lbw * Congenital malformations * preterm37 Crosstabulation

preterm37				Congenital malformations No	Congenital malformations Yes	Total
.00	lbw	.00	Count	1015	83	1098
			% within lbw	92.4%	7.6%	100.0%
			% within Congenital malformations	95.8%	92.2%	95.6%
		1.00	Count	44	7	51
			% within lbw	86.3%	13.7%	100.0%
			% within Congenital malformations	4.2%	7.8%	4.4%
	Total		Count	1059	90	1149
			% within lbw	92.2%	7.8%	100.0%
			% within Congenital malformations	100.0%	100.0%	100.0%
1.00	lbw	.00	Count	26	3	29
			% within lbw	89.7%	10.3%	100.0%
			% within Congenital malformations	31.3%	11.1%	26.4%
		1.00	Count	57	24	81
			% within lbw	70.4%	29.6%	100.0%
			% within Congenital malformations	68.7%	88.9%	73.6%
	Total		Count	83	27	110
			% within lbw	75.5%	24.5%	100.0%
			% within Congenital malformations	100.0%	100.0%	100.0%

Chi-Square Tests

preterm37		Value	df	Asymp. Sig. (2-sided)	Exact Sig. (2-sided)	Exact Sig. (1-sided)
.00	Pearson Chi-Square	2.567[b]	1	.109		
	Continuity Correction[a]	1.784	1	.182		
	Likelihood Ratio	2.154	1	.142		
	Fisher's Exact Test				.111	.097
	Linear-by-Linear Association	2.565	1	.109		
	N of Valid Cases	1149				
1.00	Pearson Chi-Square	4.288[c]	1	.038		
	Continuity Correction[a]	3.310	1	.069		
	Likelihood Ratio	4.866	1	.027		
	Fisher's Exact Test				.045	.030
	Linear-by-Linear Association	4.249	1	.039		
	N of Valid Cases	110				

a. Computed only for a 2x2 table

b. 1 cells (25.0%) have expected count less than 5. The minimum expected count is 3.99.

c. 0 cells (.0%) have expected count less than 5. The minimum expected count is 7.12.

Figure 25A. Stratification and the Chi Square Test Output.

- CROSSTABS
- /TABLES=lbw by malformations by preterm37
- /FORMAT=AVALUE TABLES
- /STATISTIC=CHISQ RISK CMH(1)
- /CELLS=COUNT ROW COLUMN
- /COUNT ROUND CELL.

Risk Estimate				
			95% Confidence Interval	
preterm37		Value	Lower	Upper
.00	Odds Ratio for lbw (.00 / 1.00)	1.946	.850	4.454
	For cohort Congenital malformations = No	1.071	.959	1.197
	For cohort Congenital malformations = Yes	.551	.268	1.130
	N of Valid Cases	1149		
1.00	Odds Ratio for lbw (.00 / 1.00)	3.649	1.008	13.213
	For cohort Congenital malformations = No	1.274	1.056	1.537
	For cohort Congenital malformations = Yes	.349	.114	1.073
	N of Valid Cases	110		

Tests of Homogeneity of the Odds Ratio			
	Chi-Squared	df	Asymp. Sig. (2-sided)
Breslow-Day	.691	1	.406
Tarone's	.658	1	.417

Tests of Conditional Independence			
	Chi-Squared	df	Asymp. Sig. (2-sided)
Cochran's	6.790	1	.009
Mantel-Haenszel	5.839	1	.016

Under the conditional independence assumption, Cochran's statistic is asymptotically distributed as a 1 df chi-squared distribution, only if the number of strata is fixed, while the Mantel-Haenszel statistic is always asymptotically distributed as a 1 df chi-squared distribution. Note that the continuity correction is removed from the Mantel-Haenszel statistic when the sum of the differences between the observed and the expected is 0.

Mantel-Haenszel Common Odds Ratio Estimate				
Estimate				2.505
ln(Estimate)				.918
Std. Error of ln(Estimate)				.347
Asymp. Sig. (2-sided)				.008
Asymp. 95% Confidence Interval	Common Odds Ratio	Lower Bound		1.268
		Upper Bound		4.949
	ln(Common Odds Ratio)	Lower Bound		.238
		Upper Bound		1.599

The Mantel-Haenszel common odds ratio estimate is asymptotically normally distributed under the common odds ratio of 1.000 assumption. So is the natural log of the estimate.

Figure 25B. Stratification and the Mantel-Haenszel Output.

Crosstabs

The first two tables (Figure 25A) are the stratification by preterm delivery; the first includes newborns born within term delivery, while the second includes newborns born within preterm delivery. We are able to look at each stratum separately, as well as each of their chi-square tests. Following, is another part of the output, in which the test of homogeneity of the odds ratio and the Mantel-Haenszel statistic is presented (Figure 25B). The test of homogeneity of the odds ratio (Breslow-Day test) is not statistically significant (p = 0.41), meaning we did not reject the null hypothesis of homogeneity of the two ORs. When looking at the last table of Figure 25B, we can notice that the Mantel-Haenszel statistic is significant (p = 0.016) and the adjusted OR is 2.51 95% CI 1.27–4.95.

The crude OR (Figure 22) estimates the risk for LBW of infants with congenital malformations when compared with infants with no congenital malformations. The risk is found to be 3.72 (95% CI 2.35–5.89, p < 0.001), as shown in Figure 22. However, the adjusted OR for LBW is slightly lower, meaning that even after controlling for preterm delivery, congenital malformation is still a risk factor for LBW.

The Mantel-Haenszel procedure is an important statistical procedure that tests the possibility of confounding; however, if the homogeneity test is significant (p < 0.05), the adjusted statistic cannot be used since we are facing an interaction or an effect modification.

Multiple Logistic Regression Model

Stratification works well only in situations in which there is only one confounder. However, usually in perinatology there are many potential confounders or risk factors that are associated with the dependent variable (outcome) [9–11]. In such a case, a multivariable analysis should be applied, which will enable determination of the independent contribution of each of the risk factors. The type of multivariable analysis depends on the outcome variable type. If the outcome variable is continuous, multiple linear regression would be the suitable model to use, although in the case of a dichotomous dependent variable or outcome, the logistic regression model should be applied, for instance, congenital malformations (yes/no) [10].

To illustrate how to perform and interpret multiple logistic regression we will use the previous example in which the outcome variable is LBW and the two risk factors are preterm delivery and congenital malformations. The result of the stratification and the Mantel-Haenszel statistic is the adjusted OR of congenital malformations, while controlling for preterm delivery. Moreover, we can perform another Mantel-Haenszel procedure in which the result will be an adjusted OR of preterm delivery while controlling for congenital malformations (stratification by congenital malformations). However, when using multiple logistic regression the results will include both of the adjusted ORs (for congenital malformations and preterm delivery).

Before performing multiple logistic regression a few rules should be emphasized [2, 10]. These rules concern the type of variables that are included in the model, in addition to the number of variables. When the dependent variable is dichotomous or binary, it is better if the format is 0/1 and not another format, such as 1/2. The latest SPSS versions recode these values to the format of 0/1, which will also be reported in the output explaining the way it was done (1 → 0; 2→ 1). The disadvantage of this method is that we cannot decide how to code the groups ourselves (which group will be coded as 1), since this decision will influence the way the ORs will be calculated. For example, if we are to perform a logistic regression for the outcome of LBW, we will code newborns with LBW as 1, and newborns with normal weight as 0. By doing so, the ORs in this model will be calculated for the risk of LBW, while being compared to normal birth weight, and not the other way around.

With regard to the independent variables (covariates) or the risk factors, the variables can be either continuous, dichotomous (yes/no), or categorical. We can enter the first two types of variables in the model in their original format. However, categorical variables with three or more groups should be entered in the model as dummy variables and not in their original format. As far as the number of covariates, the ratio of at least ten outcomes per independent variable is acceptable [9–11].

In order to perform a logistic regression, do as the following [1–3]:

- Analyze>Regression >Binary Logistic…

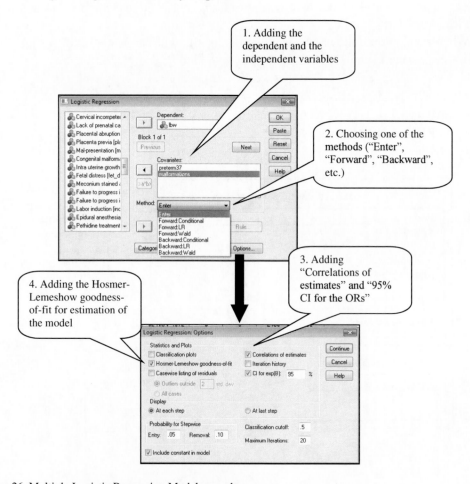

Figure 26. Multiple Logistic Regression Model procedure.

First, we will add the dependent variable (LBW) and the independent variables (preterm delivery and congenital malformations) (Figure 26, 1). Then we will choose the "Enter" method (Figure 26, 2), which forces the computer to include all the variables in the model. It is also possible to choose methods other than "Enter", such as "Forward" or "Backward" eliminations. These methods can be useful if we would like the computer to choose the included variables in this model. In most cases, we are interested in controlling for potential confounders, and should avoid using methods other than "Enter".

Next, click on "options", which will open the second screen shown in Figure 26, 2. There, check the confidence intervals and the estimation of correlations between variables included in the model (Figure 26, 3). By checking the "Correlations of estimates" we examine the correlation between covariates that are included in the model (multicollinearity). Try to avoid a high correlation between variables, because when two variables are highly correlated it is impossible for the model to identify the independent contribution of each of them. We can also add the Hosmer-Lemeshow goodness-of-fit (Figure 26, 4). Goodness-of-fit statistics are a measurement of how well an explanatory model predicts the outcome. This statistic compares the estimated to observed likelihood of outcome in the study. In a well-fitting model, the estimated likelihood will be close to that observed and the p value will not be significant (p > 0.05).

When running the following syntax, an output file will be created. Most of the output tables are shown in Figure 27A,B,C.

- LOGISTIC REGRESSION lbw
- /METHOD=ENTER preterm37 malformations
- /PRINT=GOODFIT CORR CI(95)
- /CRITERIA=PIN(.05) POUT(.10) ITERATE(20) CUT(.5).

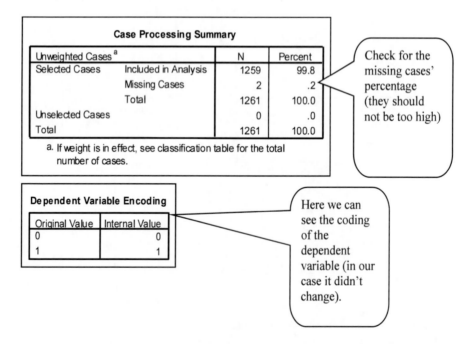

Figure 27A. Part A of the Logistic Regression Model Output—Case Processing and the Dependent Variable.

Logistic Regression

In the first table of the Logistic Regresstion Model Output (Figure 27A) there is information about the number of participants included in the analysis and the missing cases percentage. Note that the percentage of missing cases is relatively low (2%). In cases of high percentages of missing cases, we need to compare the participants who were included in the analysis to the participants who were not. This comparison is done to indicate whether there is a selection bias [8]. The next table informs us about the recoding of the dependent variable; in our example the values remain the same because the original values were 0/1.

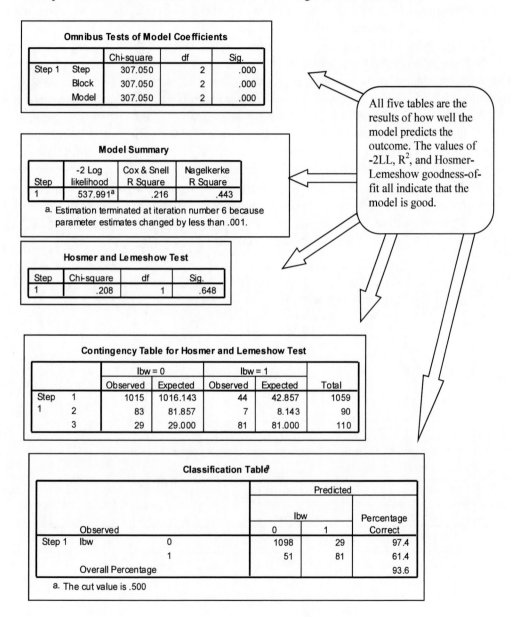

Omnibus Tests of Model Coefficients

		Chi-square	df	Sig.
Step 1	Step	307.050	2	.000
	Block	307.050	2	.000
	Model	307.050	2	.000

Model Summary

Step	-2 Log likelihood	Cox & Snell R Square	Nagelkerke R Square
1	537.991ª	.216	.443

a. Estimation terminated at iteration number 6 because parameter estimates changed by less than .001.

Hosmer and Lemeshow Test

Step	Chi-square	df	Sig.
1	.208	1	.648

Contingency Table for Hosmer and Lemeshow Test

		lbw = 0 Observed	lbw = 0 Expected	lbw = 1 Observed	lbw = 1 Expected	Total
Step 1	1	1015	1016.143	44	42.857	1059
	2	83	81.857	7	8.143	90
	3	29	29.000	81	81.000	110

Classification Tableª

			Predicted lbw 0	Predicted lbw 1	Percentage Correct
	Observed				
Step 1	lbw	0	1098	29	97.4
		1	51	81	61.4
	Overall Percentage					93.6

a. The cut value is .500

All five tables are the results of how well the model predicts the outcome. The values of -2LL, R^2, and Hosmer-Lemeshow goodness-of-fit all indicate that the model is good.

Figure 27B. Part B of the Logistic Regression Model Output—Goodness-of-Fit.

Block 1: Method = Enter

The second part of the Logistic Regression Output (Figure 27B) presents information about the goodness-of-fit statistics. These statistics are a measurement of how well an explanatory model predicts the outcome. When looking at the -2LL and the Nagelkerke R square, notice that 44% of the variance of the dependent variable (LBW) can be explained due to the covariates included in the model (preterm delivery and congenital malformations). The Hosmer-Lemeshow goodness-of-fit is not statistically significant; in addition, according to the classification table there is a total prediction of 93.6%. In conclusion, according to all the statistics above, the model goodness-of-fit is fine.

The third part of the Logistic Regresstion Output (Figure 27C) depicts information regarding the relationship between each of the independent variables (covariate) with the dependent variable. The most important results are the adjusted ORs and their 95% CIs. According to the first table (Figure 27C), infants born with congenital malformations are at a 2.4-fold risk (OR=2.4 95% CI 1.2–4.5) for LBW compared to infants without congenital malformations. Also, the risk for LBW of infants born in preterm delivery is 55.5-fold greater compared to infants born in term delivery. Both of these risks are adjusted for the other. In fact, the results of the stratification and the Mantel-Haenszel statistic, which we performed previously, are very similar to the adjusted OR originating from the logistic regression model. One of the important advantages of the regression model is being able to control for several variables at the same time. When several independent variables are included in the model, pay attention to the sample size, hence a sufficient number of LBW infants.

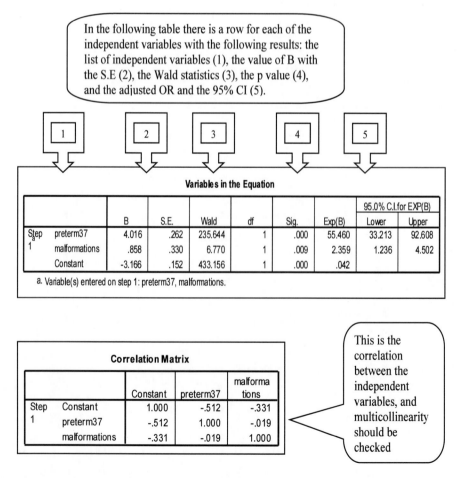

In the following table there is a row for each of the independent variables with the following results: the list of independent variables (1), the value of B with the S.E (2), the Wald statistics (3), the p value (4), and the adjusted OR and the 95% CI (5).

Variables in the Equation

		B	S.E.	Wald	df	Sig.	Exp(B)	95.0% C.I.for EXP(B) Lower	Upper
Step 1[a]	preterm37	4.016	.262	235.644	1	.000	55.460	33.213	92.608
	malformations	.858	.330	6.770	1	.009	2.359	1.236	4.502
	Constant	-3.166	.152	433.156	1	.000	.042		

a. Variable(s) entered on step 1: preterm37, malformations.

Correlation Matrix

		Constant	preterm37	malforma tions
Step 1	Constant	1.000	-.512	-.331
	preterm37	-.512	1.000	-.019
	malformations	-.331	-.019	1.000

This is the correlation between the independent variables, and multicollinearity should be checked

Figure 27C. Part C of the Logistic Regression Model Output—The Relationship between the Independent Variables and the Dependent Variable.

In the last table (Figure 27C) there is information about the correlations between the independent variables. Try to avoid a situation of high correlation between covariates included in the model (multicollinearity). In the case of a high correlation, change the model, for example, by removing one of the variables [9–11].

SUMMARY

Although performing data analysis with SPSS® for Windows would be considered relatively friendly and simple, in the case of a perinatal study we should be very careful in the process of choosing a suitable statistical test.

Start with the descriptive statistics followed by the bivariable analysis; perform the multivariable analysis only at the end of the process.

In the field of perinatal epidemiology, the multivariable analysis models are a very important tool due to their ability to control for potential confounders. However, by performing all of the data analysis steps mentioned in this chapter, one will have better knowledge of the data, hence a better statistical analysis resulting in an improved ability to reach correct conclusions.

REFERENCES

[1]   *SPSS for Windows, 14.0: User's guide.* Chicago: SPSS Inc.; 2005.

[2]   Field A. *Discovering statistics using SPSS for windows. 2nd ed.* London: SAGE Publications; 2005.

[3]   Landau S, Everitt BS. *A Handbook of Statistical Analysis using SPSS.* Boca Raton, FL: Chapman & Hall/CRC Press; 2004.

[4]   Stevens J. *Statistical analysis of epidemiology data. 2nd ed.* New York: Oxford University Press; 1996.

[5]   Woodward M. *Epidemiology study design and data analysis. 2nd ed.* Boca Raton, FL: Chapman & Hall/CRC Press; 2005.

[6]   Lilienfeld DE, Stolley PD. *Foundations of Epidemiology. 3rd ed.* New York: Oxford University Press; 1994.

[7]   Kelsey JL, Whittemore AS, Evans AS, Thompson WD. *Methods in Observational Epidemiology. 2nd ed.* New York: Oxford University Press; 1996.

[8]   Szklo M, Nieto FJ. *Epidemiology: beyond the basics. 2nd ed.* Sudbury, MA: Jones and Bartlett Publishers; 2007.

[9]   Stevens J. *Applied multivariate statistics for the social sciences.* Mahwah, NJ: Lawrence Erlbaum Associates, Inc.; 2001.

[10]   Hosmer DW, Lemeshow S. *Applied logistic regression.* New York: John Wiley & Sons, Inc.; 1989.

[11]   Katz MH. *Multivariable analysis: a practical guide for clinicians. 2nd ed.* New York: Cambridge University Press; 2006.

In: Handbook of Methodological Concepts in Perinatal Medicine   ISBN: 978-1-62081-252-5
Editor: Eyal Sheiner   © 2013 Nova Science Publishers, Inc.

Chapter 9

META-ANALYSES

Hairong Xu [*] *and William D. Fraser*

Department of Obstetrics and Gynecology, Hôpital Sainte-Justine,
Université de Montréal, QC, Canada

DEFINITION

Meta-Analysis: A study which combines the results of several studies that address a set of related research hypotheses.

INTRODUCTION

Clinicians are increasingly required to guide their practice based on the best available evidence. Synthesis of the available evidence therefore remains essential for good clinical practice. One of important approaches to handling a vast array of data is systematic review. A systematic review is a form of research that provides a summary of medical reports, using explicit methods to search, critically appraise and synthesize the published or unpublished evidence concerning a specific clinical question. Quantitative systematic review, or meta-analysis, combine different studies to produce an overall effect estimate of a specific treatment using explicit statistical techniques. The role of systematic review and meta-analysis has been increasingly endorsed in evidence-based decision making. The present chapter provides an overview of basic and quantitative methods and issues needed to be considered for the conduct of meta-analysis.

---

[*] Hairong Xu, MD, PhD, Department of Obstetrics and Gynecology and Social and Preventive Medicine, Université de Montréal hairongxx@yahoo.ca.

HISTORY OF META-ANALYSIS

In 1904, Karl Pearson - a pioneering biostatistician, was probably the first to use formal techniques to combine data from different studies when investigating the preventive effect of serum inoculations against enteric fever. [1] Although meta-analysis is widely used in epidemiology and evidence-based medicine today, a meta-analysis of a medical treatment was not published until 1955. In 1976, the psychologist Gene Class first introduced the term 'meta-analysis' in a paper entitled 'primary, secondary, and meta-analysis of research'. [2] In the 1980s, meta analysis became more popular in medicine, in particular in the clinical trials of cardiovascular disease, oncology, and perinatal care.

In the 1980s, the Oxford Database of Perinatal Trials (ODPT) was founded and initially sought to create a registry of perinatal trials to "provide a resource for reviews of the safety and efficacy of interventions used in perinatal care". [3,4] In 1993, the Cochrane Pregnancy and Childbirth Database (CCPC) was published by reissuing the systematic reviews contained in the ODPT. [5] With the success of CCPC, the Cochrane Collaboration - an international network of health care professionals who prepare and regularly update systematic reviews ('Cochrane Reviews') - was established to facilitate the conduct of meta analysis in all fields of health care. [6] Since 1996, systematic reviews prepared and maintained through the Cochrane Collaboration have been published in The Cochrane Library. The Cochrane Database of Systematic Reviews, a component of the Cochrane Library, is periodically updated by professionals as more information becomes available and in response to comments and criticism.

STUDY IDENTIFICATION

Before commencing a meta-analysis, the first step is to determine 'what is your research question', including the definition of the principal exposure of interest and the outcome(s). For instance, one may be interested in investigating the effects of calcium supplementation during pregnancy (exposure) on the risk of preeclampsia (outcome). Then, a difficult but crucial task is to identify studies that are relevant to addressing the question. The reviewer must decide which type of study design should be included. For instance, one may decide to include only randomized trials or all relevant studies, including both observational studies and clinical trials. This decision will depend on the exposure under investigation and potential for bias in nonrandomized studies. A search of computerized databases (e.g. MEDLINE, PUBMED) may provide a reasonable start, but is often insufficient because not all studies are included in such databases. Some studies, particularly ones with negative results, may go unpublished and some may be published but only as abstracts or in journals not captured in electronic databases. One should manually search through references of each identified report in order to identify all relevant studies. In addition, databases that include information on graduate study theses may yield additional unpublished studies. One may also contact researchers who are experts in the field to see if they are aware of any unpublished data on such topics. In the end, it should be realized that the results may be biased due to systematic failure of other investigators to publish or report certain data (e.g. null results). Restricting the analysis to include only published data may aggravate such bias.

STUDY QUALITY

The validity of systematic reviews or meta-analyses depends heavily on the validity of the individual studies included. In some sense, the quantitative methods used to pool the results from several studies in a meta-analysis is of less importance than the qualitative methods employed to assess which studies should be aggregated.

To date, several approaches have been developed for assessing study quality, including the validity framework by Cook and Campbell, [7] scales and checklists by Moher *et al.* [8] and Deeks *et al.* [9] Although quality assessment scales may provide an overall estimate of quality, the validity of these scales has been questioned. It has been noted that most scales have been developed in an arbitrary fashion and serve better to evaluate the adequacy of reporting of a study rather than the quality of design and conduct of the study. The scales differ considerably in terms of dimensions covered, size, complexity and the weight assigned to the key domains most relevant to the control of bias such as randomization, blinding, and loss to follow up. In order to assess whether the types of scales used for assessing the quality of trials affects the conclusions of meta-analytic studies, Jüni *et al.* repeated a published meta analysis using different quality assessment scales. [10] The result indicated that none of the 25 scales yielded a statistically significant association between summary scores and effect sizes, and the effect size either increased or decreased with increasing trial quality depending on the scales used. The authors concluded that although the use of a summary score to identify trials of high quality is problematic, the relevant methodological aspects (e.g. concealment of treatment allocation, blinding of outcome assessment or double blinding, and handling of withdrawals and dropouts) should be always identified a priori, and assessed individually. [10] Greenland also pointed out that quality dimensions are highly application specific and therefore hard to measure from published information and the use of quality scores to weight studies in a meta-analysis could produce biased effect estimates. [11]

There appears to be little consensus concerning the optimum approach to dealing with study quality in meta-analysis. However, there is general agreement that a critical evaluation of studies included in the meta-analysis is essential for the interpretation of the results. Efforts to standardize the unbiased conduct and reporting of both randomized trials and meta-analyses should be enhanced.

Definition of Outcome Measures

Outcome measures in meta-analysis include measures such as odds ratio (OR), relative risk (RR), risk difference (RD), number needed to treat (NNT), mean difference, and standardized mean difference. Before combining the studies, one needs to choose a measure to use, based on consideration of whether it is statistically appropriate and convenient to work with, and whether it is clinically meaningful. For example, 'Number needed to treat' has been increasingly used in reporting clinical trials as it may provide a more useful and meaningful approach for clinical decision making. If the outcome of interest is rare, one may ignore the distinctions between odds ratios and rate ratios. However, this distinction can be important when studying outcomes that are frequent, especially in case-control design and analysis. Studies can be combined directly using the reported measures in each study if each study uses the same scale to measure the same parameter. Otherwise, it is common practice to transform data into the same standardized scale if different scales are used in each study if such transformation is possible.

EXPRESSING THE EFFECTS ACROSS STUDIES (FIXED AND RANDOM EFFECTS MODELS)

The decision as to whether to utilize a statistical technique to summarize the effects across studies is based on several considerations, including statistical heterogeneity and clinical heterogeneity.

These questions are addressed in more detail in the following section. The use of standard univariate fixed- and random-effects models in meta-analysis has become well known in the last 20 years. A fixed effects model to combine treatment effects assumes no heterogeneity between studies and assumes that the true treatment effect is the same in all studies. The

overall treatment effect then is estimated as a weighted average- $\hat{\theta} = \dfrac{\sum_{i=1}^{k} w_i \hat{\theta}_i}{\sum_{i=1}^{k} w_i}$, where $\hat{\theta}_i$ is

observed effect estimate in ith study, k is the number of studies included in the meta-analysis, w_i is the weight of the ith study ($w_i = 1/v_i$). The $\hat{\theta}_i$ is assumed to have an approximate normal distribution of $N(\theta, v_i)$. Other fixed effect methods have been developed to combine the effect estimates (e.g. odds ratios) including Mantel-Haenszel method, [12] Peto's method [13] and maximum likelihood techniques [14].

Compared to the fixed effect model, the random effects model assumes that the effects between studies are different and vary at random. An additional variance component which accounts for the between study variance ($\sigma^2{}_B$) is therefore added in random effects models to incorporate heterogeneity. The overall random effects estimate is given by

$\hat{\theta} = \dfrac{\sum_{i=1}^{k} w_i^{*} \hat{\theta}_i}{\sum_{i=1}^{k} w_i^{*}}$, where $w_i^{*} = 1/(v_i + \hat{\sigma}_B{}^2)$, $\hat{\theta}_i$ estimates the individual treatment effects

with a distribution of $N(\theta_i, v_i)$, and the true treatment effects in each study θ_i (random effects) is assumed to have a distribution of $N(\theta, \sigma^2{}_B)$. Generally, the between study variance ($\sigma^2{}_B$) can be estimated using either a moment estimate (weighted or unweighted least square) or maximum or restricted maximum likelihood methods. [15,16,17] Likelihood based approaches [15] yield, in general, wider confidence intervals than those generated with the standard random effects models (e.g. the approach of DerSimonian and Laird). [16]

It is worth noting that the confidence intervals for point estimates of treatment effects derived from a random effects model are wider than those from the corresponding fixed effect model. Different analytical models may lead to the different, or even opposite conclusions. [17-19] There is much debate on policies for choosing fixed versus random effects models. [17,20,21] Some researchers have advocated the use of random effects model even if there is no evidence of statistical heterogeneity. [22] As fixed and random effects models address